The Hospital at the End of the World

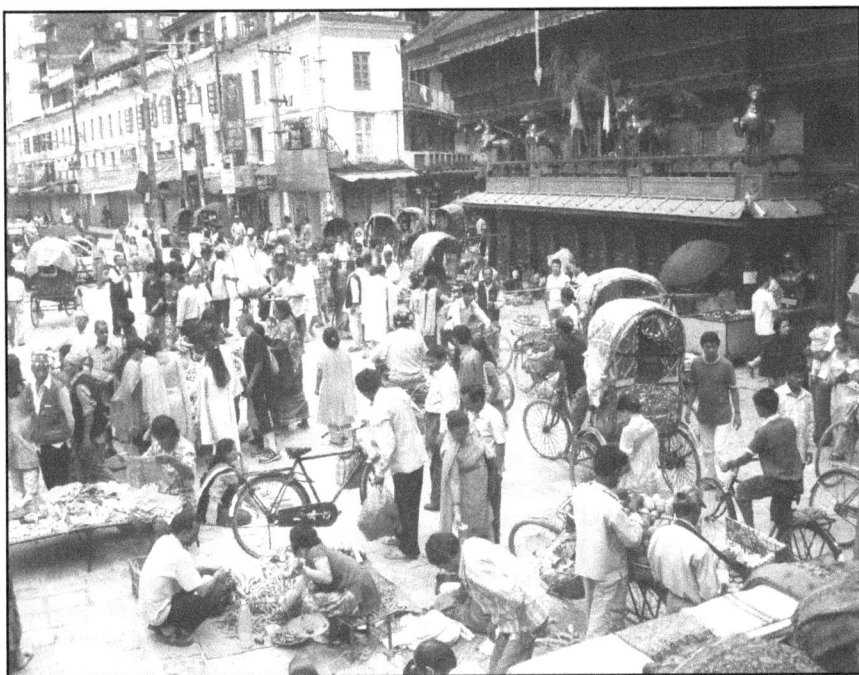

Medical stories from a place far off the beaten path of twenty-first-century medicine. A front row seat with Christian medical missionaries in the foothills of the Himalayas

Joe Niemczura, RN, MS

Plain View Press
1011 W. 34th Street, Suite 260
Austin, TX 78705

www.plainviewpress.net

ISBN: 978-0-911051-37-7
Library of Congress Number: 2009927910

Photographs on the cover and throughout the book are by the author.

Photo on title page: Indra Chowk in Old Kathmandu. Large crowds of people going about their business. This photo conveys the population density of urban Nepal, and the reliance on foot-powered transportation, very striking to a newcomer to the country. Note the rickshaws and vegetable sellers.

Introduction

This book uses a number of words from the Nepali language which are used daily among the English-speaking missionaries in Nepal. The glossary of Nepali terms at the end of the book defines all such words for the reader's convenience.

Gentle reader: This book is not for the casual armchair traveler. Nepal has wonderful people as well as colorful local customs and scenery, but if you expect to read about these things, you should find some other book.

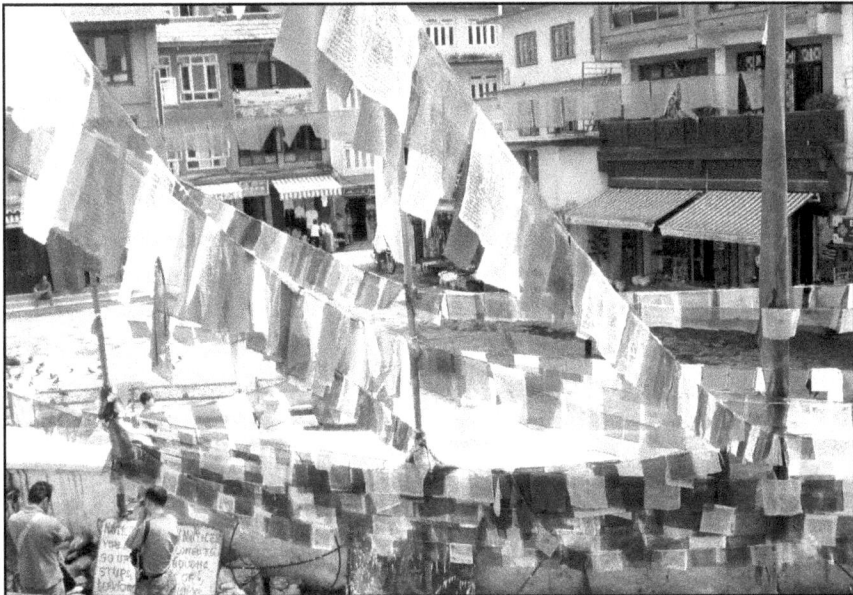

At Boudhanath, looking down from the second level onto the Kora track below, a profusion of prayer flags. In the corners of the *stupa* are spaces where devout Buddhists practice ritual prostration, aligning their *chakras*, as a form of meditation.

Dedication

To my brother Peter – I miss your advice and sense of humor. Stop laughing at me from wherever you are. I know I will see you again, hopefully not soon.

To Amy and Julie – the best daughters I could have asked for, and the best teachers I ever had. "When you look for happiness on life's journey, may you always find it."

To Mary – You were the best travel companion ever, and the best friend of my entire life. I still wish that last train had been headed down a different set of tracks.

And finally – to the mothers of sick or injured children everywhere.

Contents

The Bubble

The Non-Governmental Organization that brought me to Nepal told me the owner of the Salome Guest House would meet me at the airport and that he was reliable. I exchanged my dollars for rupees, got my visa, collected my eight boxes of baggage, cleared customs, and walked down the exit corridor. Around the corner was a mob of clamoring cab drivers pounding on a chain-link fence at the terminal to get the attention of potential customers. Sure enough, one guy was holding a printout of my photo – he must be the one! Eight porters grabbed my boxes before I could stop them, forming a small parade to the car. We pushed through the crowd and loaded the boxes in to the trunk. The driver stood by as I had a brief dispute with the porters about payment. In my pocket there was seventy-thousand rupees, but the smallest bill was a five-hundred rupee note. I did not want to spend four-thousand rupees on five minute's work. I gave them a five-hundred rupee note, just one, and told them to share it. They were slapping on the windows of the car as we pulled out.

"I could have used some help with those porters," I said to the driver as we got moving. He was expressionless as he kept his eyes on the road.

"You did okay." He shifted into second gear and said, "You stayed calm, that's the main thing. It's not up to me how much money you spend on porters."

He thought for a moment, adding, "And besides, I have to come back here tomorrow. I don't like to draw attention to myself at the airport."

I joined him in looking straight ahead as we inched through a crowd of people waiting right at the airport gates.

Before I could think about what he said, we turned onto the main road, and I could have reached out the window to touch a funeral procession on foot headed toward God-knows-where. A shrouded body on a white bamboo litter was carried on the shoulders of four sweating pallbearers with a trailing group of thirty people in pairs on foot behind. We swerved to avoid the women squatting by charcoal fires to cook corn on the cob by the side of the road. For a moment, five dark-skinned men wearing blue plaid skirts and blue turbans rode alongside us on bicycles, balancing baskets of apples big as hula hoops. We passed a construction crew balancing pans of wet concrete on their heads as they climbed up a ladder to pour the new floor of a building.

The car slowly zigzagged around piles of gravel, then bricks, then debris blocking the road nearby. Women wearing red carried woven bamboo baskets full of vegetables on their backs using a tumpline around their forehead. There were clumps of other women in colorful *saris* which billowed in the breeze, every shade of red and purple. Signs in Sanskrit receded into the distance before they could be read. We made sudden lurching stops so as not to go airborne when the pavement ended altogether for short stretches. Cows stood in the street next to an open-air market where men sold wristwatches, shoes, plastic backpacks, Barbie dolls and plastic basins of various sizes.

The cloudy stench of diesel exhaust fumes filled my nose. We saw a green oasis of serenity which turned out to be a military checkpoint with razor wire outside the royal palace. We passed rusting, silvery *tuk-tuks*, no bigger than a mini pickup, loaded with people packed in like sardines, three or four men standing on each back bumper. Loose dogs rooted through piles of rotting trash on street. Squadrons of up to twenty motorcycles roared by, a cacophony of horns – all traffic driving on left, line of taxis queuing for fuel. A bridge was next. Down the embankment in the flood zone of the river was a sign that said "U.N. Refugee Camp." Behind it, stretching off for a kilometer or so, were two parallel rows of tents made of tattered blue tarp. In the river itself, a bloated dead cow was stuck on a sandbar. Three boys waded nearby. On the bridge, a naked man – a *sadhu* perhaps – was defecating on the sidewalk as pedestrians veered around him. Sheer masses of humanity. Chaos. I looked at a clock and realized that *only thirty minutes had passed.* There were eighty-four days to go.

I wondered what they would say at the University if they saw me now. And it had not even begun. It was only two days since I closed my office door in Honolulu for the last time for three months. I always wanted to work in a foreign culture, and now I was doing it. *Seven months of planning. Was I ready? Fantasy meets reality.*

Soon the car slowed as it crept down a dusty unpaved alley with high stucco walls on either side, broken glass embedded in the top. We stopped at a gate made of blue corrugated steel which squealed with rust as the driver opened it. As we unloaded my seven boxes of textbooks, I saw that the yard was an oasis of green, the first stop on my journey. The Guest House was red brick with a plaster statue of Ganesh embedded under the eaves. Up the stairs and inside, it was cool and quiet. I said *Namaste* to the *Didi*. The room was very simple but clean.

A dog barked incessantly all night and I lay awake thinking about the Bubble. The bubble is an imaginary envelope with invisible boundaries. It's the set of preconceived notions that people take with them when they travel, and for this trip I wanted to get beyond sightseeing, get beyond the usual superficialities that provide a comfort zone. *I was out of the Bubble now.*

The next morning I was up at five, reminding myself it was Wednesday. I walked through the streets of Patan, impatient to get some exercise after two days of flying and eating airport food. The skies were overcast. The first surprise was to see crowds of people, already out and about, shoulder-to-shoulder, hundreds of people, then around a corner to see hundreds more. *And not another westerner in sight.* The streets were narrow and unpaved and the sewer stank where they were working on it. A meat market displayed a neat row of goat's heads on a greasy table, hide scraped clean of hair, horns and blue eyes intact. My hand was in my pocket, gripping my wallet as I walked. Many temples and shrines, with votive candles, door lintels smeared with red paste.

I found Patan Durbar Square, a jumble of five-hundred-year-old temples on a brick plaza, and wandered through it, pausing to watch a street performer as he showed the audience his collection of snakes, holding them up by the tail and prodding them with a stick. Each snake seemed eager to get back in the wooden box after it was handled. I bought some milky Nepali tea and sat on the steps at one end of the square while I drank it. The day was another blur of chaotic sights and sounds, interrupted only by the time I spent in the Museum at the Square, looking at ancient metal sculpture in an oasis of serenity. I was proud that I managed not to get lost. I slept better that night, out of sheer exhaustion.

At six Thursday morning, the Buck arrived but was too ungainly to get down the alley to the Salome where I was staying so the driver sent a messenger. Like a procession of ants we carried my boxes to the wider street. Then I climbed aboard, claiming a window seat. The Buck was the vehicle operated by United Missions to Nepal (UMN) as a shuttle. It carried cargo as well as people. This cross between bus and truck is compressed into "Buck." The steering wheel was on the right, since traffic was on the left. Like all buses in Nepal, the driver had an assistant. The man who rode "shotgun" would help the driver park, back up when needed and manage other chores. Each time the Buck slowed to go through a town, the shotgun stood in the open doorway, like a train conductor. The Buck was the only vehicle I saw in Nepal that lacked a plastic Ganesh - the Hindu God known as the Remover of Obstacles - on the dash. I supposed this was a small concession to the Christian NGO that owned it. Unlike the public buses, nobody rode on the roof of the Buck, and there were no critters on board. That day we loaded some refrigerated blood and some chemotherapy drugs to deliver to the hospital in Bharatpur located along the way, a piece of equipment that had been repaired in Kathmandu, my suitcase, and of course my seven boxes of books, a little battered but intact.

The Kathmandu Valley is a huge bowl, and the bus trip to Tansen started with a climb up to the rim – as if we were an insect trying to climb out of a soup dish. After we reached the rim for the next two hours we descended continuously, one hairpin turn after another. Then a drive through the *Terai*, the large flat plain that extends along the southern border with India. I could feel myself getting further and further away. *Away from.... everything.* My eyes were glued to the window. After passing many flat rice-paddies, we began a two-hour ride up a dusty, winding mountain road with a looming cliff on the inside and a precipice on the other side. There was no guardrail, and we slowed to thread recent wheel tracks where the road had been filled in after recent landslides. On the bus ahead of us, there were passengers on the roof, and I watched the Shotgun of that bus as he climbed up to the roof and back down, while the bus was in motion. *Neat trick.* We came around a corner in the road and narrowly missed mowing down a dozen school children near a small hamlet. This made me a bit anxious but nobody else was concerned.

Finally we came to the town of Tansen, driving slowly through it. The gate to the hospital is a row of steel bars that filled a gap in an eight-foot-high cement wall. The gate was partly blocked by a pile of gravel near a cement mixer. The dust from the Buck still hung in the air as a crew of men in light blue uniforms carried my boxes of books to a storeroom. The remaining equipment was whisked away.

I was in Tansen, four days after I left Honolulu.

At first glance the hospital reminded me of a rundown factory I once saw from the window of a train passing through Milwaukee. The sign announcing the hospital was pockmarked with rust. A huge hole in the ground on the street side marked the location of the future new Emergency Room (ER) and garage. Piles of steel reinforcement bars, like huge spaghetti, waited to be shaped for concrete pilings. Rusting pieces of equipment stood in the open – a broken stretcher, an empty metal cabinet, an old stainless steel autoclave machine. A pall of smoke that smelled of burning plastic hung in the air. The brick walls of the hospital were streaked with lime and needed mortar in the chinks. Window moldings needed painting. Over each window was a metal grid, and I could see fifty-five gallon steel drums spaced on the roof, on little platforms perched over the corrugated tin. *Was I really going to spend my summer working inside this place?*

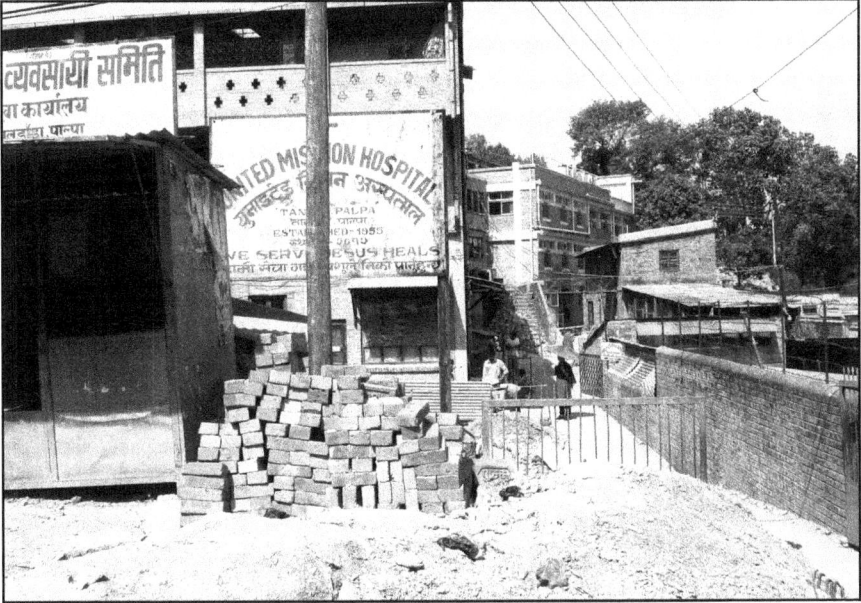

View of "lower gate" at Mission Hospital. Not the most welcoming of all the possible sights, but in 2007 the hospital embarked on a very ambitious construction project, to build a new ER.

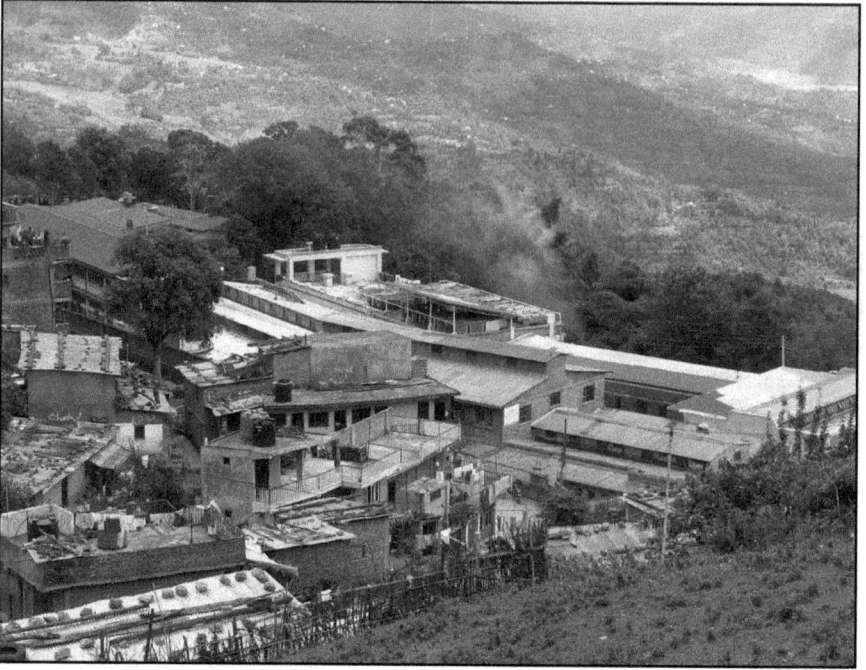

The roofs of Mission Hospital in Tansen, viewed from Partway up Shree Nagar Hill. In the foreground are the "hotels" of Shanti-town. Also visible are the sections which house the Operating Theater and Pediatrics. Staff residences were behind and to the left

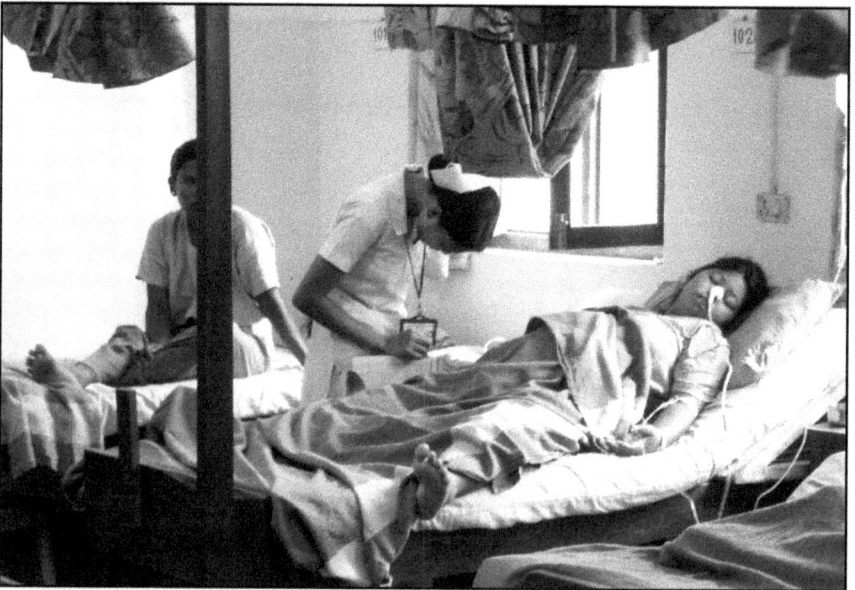

There was very little space between the beds. This lady on the Gynae Ward was one day post-op cholecystectomy.

Making a Map of the Beds

"We are giving you a thorough orientation because we think you might become a full time missionary someday." I was told.

The three-week orientation started with the Adult Medical Ward, in the oldest part of the hospital. The Medical Ward consists of a warren of rooms with no single central corridor. The walls are whitewashed brick and the floor is bare concrete. There is no glass in the windows, just mesh screen to keep out the largest insects. The doors are wooden and need paint. The medications are kept in a rolling wooden cabinet that has the distress marks of a fine antique. It has been in use since the founding of the hospital in 1952. The thermometers are the old-fashioned mercury kind; and they are kept in a special wooden box with a purple velvet lining. Forceps are soaking in alcohol in a stainless steel covered dish. The posters on the wall are in a mixture of Nepali and English. In the patient rooms, the drapes between beds do not match. The whole effect reminds me of being in a Scottish castle, or at least my fantasies of what a castle would be like if you were trying to use it for a hospital. The Medical Ward has thirty beds, and the numbering system is so confusing that on the second day I found a piece of blank paper and sketched out a crude map of the rooms, showing the location of the beds and the numbers, just so I could keep track of where individual patients are located.

May 30 was my third day. My portable alarm clock rang as the *Chowkidar* walked by, making his last rounds through the complex for the night. It was before dawn. I boiled water then added it to a pitcher with the coffee grounds. After the coffee steeped, I poured it through a wire mesh filter into my cup. It was still a bit grainy. I sipped the coffee in my apartment and scrambled some eggs. Across the way in a nearby dorm, a teakettle whistled and one of the female Nepali doctors sang a lilting Hindi song as she made tea in her apartment. Over the summer I was usually up and out before she was, but I loved to hear her sing, as it reminded me that I was in a particular time and a particular place. Later somebody told me that she probably was a Krishna devotee and the singing was part of her morning *puja* – prayers. There were five women on the junior medical staff. When they made rounds I would listen to their voices and try to figure out which one might be the singer, but I never was able to settle on just one possibility.

The night nurses hand over their patients to the oncoming day shift at "morning report," promptly at seven. I got there at six, early enough to copy down the names and numbers so I would not get lost, since report was conducted in two languages. This time I scratched my head, because the night nurses kept referring to extra room numbers I could not find on the little map I had made the day before. *What in hell?* I turned the map over a few times. *They have a system here; I just don't happen to have a clue what it is.* Soon it dawned on me that there were *thirty-nine* patients that day. Nine patients were lying on low pallets at various locations in each room to supplement the thirty in beds. I had to go look and double check because I could not believe it at first. And each patient, whether on the floor or not, had at least one relative with them. In many cases, their family member was still asleep on a bedroll *under* the patient's bed; these people were beginning to stir and some held their bedroll under their arm, preparing to leave. It was my first exposure to what I called the "Bus Station Effect" – a mass of humanity.

My impressions of foreignness were magnified by the appearance and clothes of those around me. Some of the women wore a *sari*, pink or purple, but the favorite color seemed to be blood red. I saw other women decked out in ankle-length skirts, shawls, long sleeved blouses, and a strange bulky piece of cloth wound about ten times around their waists. It made them all look pregnant, even the elderly women. The colors jarred the western eye. For example, a woman might wear red, purple and pink along with green. Some women were wearing huge golden earrings and nose rings that drooped down below their lips. *Toto, I have the feeling that we are not in Kansas anymore.*

One four-bed room on the Medical Ward was called the Critical Ward. With their Nepali accents, the doctors and nurses pronounced this *"KRIT–ti-Kull,* with the accent on the first syllable. It sounded just exotic enough to make me smile. It was not an Intensive Care Unit (ICU) with modern equipment. It was merely the room closest to the nurse's station.

At change-of-shift report, we learned that there were two patients whose oxygen saturation was running in the sixties. As soon as report was over, I quickly found the oxygen measuring device. It is called a pulse oximeter, or "pulse ox" when you are in a hurry. To use it, you put the person's finger between two clothespin-like arms, and a red light shines through that tells you how red the blood is. The redness is related to how much oxygen is in the bloodstream. Simple and elegant. If the machine indicated that the blood was turning darker, you could quantify it by assigning a percentage to the change. Anything below ninety per cent indicates trouble. Pulse ox was the most reliable machine at Mission Hospital for those occasions when we wanted to see whether a patient was deteriorating. Medical Ward owned two of them. It was the same brand we used in the US, but for some reason these devices did not seem as sturdy. They would go unreliable at random times or so it seemed.

In another room a man lay dying of tetanus – also known as lockjaw. I had never seen a person die from this before, so I drew a red star next to his name on my list. We also had a young woman suffering from diarrhea. One of the nurses told me in hushed tones that it was *Supalba,* the local term for AIDS, and the patient was a prostitute who had returned from India. *Make another red star next to this name too. Here is a woman who has been an actual slave, in real time. In my life time.* In Nepal, women are forced into prostitution. It is not a career choice. Call it what it is: sex slavery. *She was 'free' now, but serving a death sentence.*

One of our two critical patients was a thirty-year-old man with pneumonia and the other was a twenty-two-year-old woman with chronic renal failure. When I got the pulse ox, I rushed to this room first and stuck the pulse ox on my own finger. It read 97%, which was what I expected to read on myself, a healthy person. This is a rough way to see if the device is working. Then I stuck it on the fingers of our two patients, and confirmed that yes indeed, each was running in the sixties – a critically low level of oxygen in their bloodstream. In the US, these two would be in ICU on a mechanical ventilator, a machine to supplement their breathing. Here they were getting oxygen via mask, and each was breathing fast and labored. I looked around and there was no crash cart and no heart monitor. The young woman's mother was at the bedside. She was about forty years old and short – maybe five feet at best. The mother wore the outfit with the waist wrap and a shawl, even though it was about eighty-five degrees.

These two are going to die today. This thought came, divorced of sentimentality or emotion. *A simple scientific fact.* I took a gut check of my emotional reaction to the situation because it's the first step before responding. Like many people who do critical care, I use a few mental tricks to help myself stay on track.

The first approach to a critical situation is to "go into Spok mode," named after the character on the TV show Star Trek. Mister Spok is the alien who can only deal in facts. Spok has no emotion whatsoever, and many of the plots of the TV show are based on his inability to process love, hate, or ambiguity. So the first response in any emergency is factual. *Focus on the data, get the equipment, examine the patient systematically, and remain open to the situation as it presents itself.*

Sometimes in a hospital, there is advance notice that a trauma victim is coming in, which means workers have the luxury of five or ten minutes to prepare. The team assembles, roles are assigned and equipment is rechecked. Some say a quick prayer. Of course, there are many who don't do these exercises, and end up relying on alcohol or some form of escape after the event. The less said about this, the better. The visualization exercise I use the most, which really seems to work, I call "putting Little Joe to bed."

"Little Joe" is my name for my inner Child, that part of me that is still a five-year-old boy. We all have this, no matter how old we become. Kids that age might become frightened or anxious by things they saw in the world for which there was no explanation. In real life, a good parent would never allow their child to see a scary movie, or play in the street, or tell them a ghost story, or do anything that disrupted the zone of safety and love around them. To "put Little Joe to bed," I mentally pick him up, tell him I love him, and that *grownup things are now going to happen and he does not need to be around, we will tell him later what happened and he is going to be safe.* Then I mentally tuck him in and focus on the task at hand.

People who don't do health care sometimes say, "Oh, you must get hardened to it somehow." But when I use this technique I never think of it as hardening. People don't grow immune to suffering. Nurses and doctors learn that in order to be effective they need to manage their emotional reactions. Here in Tansen, I mentally put Little Joe to bed that morning. *Later we can laugh and play. Not now.*

While I was rechecking the oxygen level on our two critical patients, the doctors arrived to make rounds. The doctors went first into the room where the two patients with low oxygen were chugging away. While we were still talking about what to do, the young woman with renal failure stopped breathing. We could not feel a pulse. The doctors decided to try to revive her. As the mother stood by, we started CPR and got out the airway box. *There was no heart monitor.* We found the patient's IV line and gave epinephrine, then calcium gluconate based on the idea that her potassium was probably high due to the renal failure. We attempted to put a breathing tube in her throat and got it into place, but it did not seem to make any difference.

First ten minutes passed, then twenty. The mother stood by very quietly and watched. We could see the likelihood of success dwindling away. We ran out of things to try. When forty minutes had passed, the doctor in charge called a halt. To confirm death, the doctors listened for a heart beat and felt for a pulse. There was none. Then they got out a cotton ball, and gently touched a wisp of it to the patient's cornea. The lack of a blink was taken to be a sign of profound neurological deficit consistent with death. The doctor then matter-of-factly discussed the outcome with the mother, who did not show any signs of emotion.

The man with tetanus was not a candidate for heroic measures, and the scene was quiet when he too, died. We did have one success – the thirty-year-old man with low oxygen was given nebulized medication to open his airways, and he improved as the antibiotics kicked in to treat his pneumonia. When his fever broke he was drenched in sweat.

That night I had a dream in which I was in my first car, my canary yellow 1966 VW beetle, with my college girlfriend. We were driving through a city – maybe Boston, maybe San Francisco. The buildings were American but the street scene was pure Nepal. There were cows in the road. I was trying to drive on the left like they do in Nepal. Every time we had a near-miss, she stamped her foot on the floor, pumping the imaginary brake on the passenger's side and bracing for a crash. This part of the dream was not new, it was a part of our life together for many years. One of my brothers refused to drive with us because it made him too tense to watch us interact this way. That night, there was something new in the dream: she kept pulling the wheel, trying to get me to drive on the right like they do in Boston. I don't remember how the dream ended.

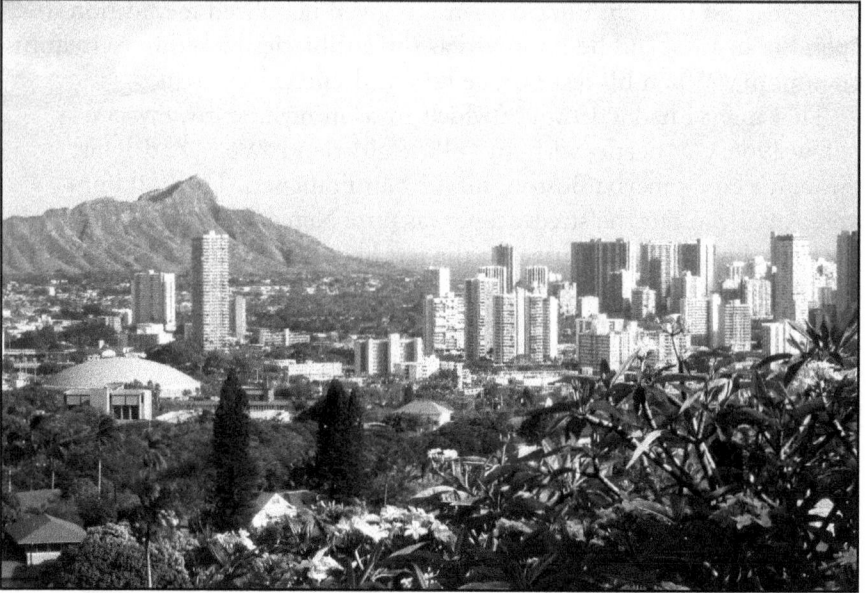

While I was away, my parents enjoyed sunrise over Diamond Head and the lights of the Waikiki Skyline. View from my front yard in Manoa, near the University. Bus # 5 is the closest route.

Leaving Honolulu

My dad is eighty-two years old and my mom is seventy-nine. When they heard I was going away for the summer, they decided to rent my apartment in Hawaii for three months. Stan and Alicia arrived two days before I left. I met them at the airport with a hug and a kiss for each and then draped a flower garland, a *lei* around their necks. "This is the traditional welcome to the Islands," I said. On the way to the apartment in Manoa, my mom said that every morning the ladies of the retirement community in Florida shared a cup of coffee by the pool.

"When I told them I was going to stay in Hawaii for three months while my son the University Professor did Humanitarian work in Nepal, everyone was impressed. I got a lot of mileage out of you already." As she said this, Alicia looked out the car window at the Pacific Ocean and beamed.

There were long silences from my dad but I took them for granted because he is hard of hearing. He tends to shout when he says anything at all. I still sometimes cringe the way I did when I was eight. My mom seems to be used to the shouting after fifty-six years of marriage. "Ever since you were a kid I told you to ignore him, he's been partly deaf since nineteen-forty-five." I brought their baggage up the steps to the apartment. The first thing my dad unpacked was the laptop, and he took over the walk-in closet for his computer room. He anxiously checked to see whether he could access the internet using my landlord's Wi-Fi network. Fortunately, he could get online with no problem. Then he relaxed a bit. From his luggage he found a bag of M & Ms. He poured out a few and ate them, one at a time, while he finished unpacking.

I drove my parents to the city bus office in Kalihi, an urban neighborhood well away from Waikiki. Tourists have no reason to go to Kalihi. We bought two bus passes so Mom and Dad would not have to drive through downtown traffic. As long as I could remember, my dad was busy with some project or another, and my brothers and I served as his inexpensive private labor pool. That is how he taught us carpentry, plumbing, sheetrock, electrical wiring, auto repair, welding, and masonry. In retirement we all worried that he would die of boredom. Despite spending time on the computer, he needed a project. As we drove to the airport for my departure, he shouted to me that he had an idea to pass the time – his goal was to ride every bus route in the Honolulu system at least once. He already had the map of the system, and he would go back to the Bus Headquarters in Kalihi and stock up on the individual route schedules. In the rearview mirror I could see my mom in the back seat mouthing the words, "He's crazy," and wagging her eyes.

"Where did you get that idea? The bus system does not give frequent flyer miles if that is what you are after," I said in a voice loud enough for him to hear. Then in a resigned tone, "You'll certainly see a part of Oahu most tourists don't see." What I did not tell him was that this plan was stunning in its futile grandiosity and I had to admire the imagination that would generate such an audacious undertaking. When my dad gets the idea for a project, he will stick with it to the end. *I worry when I find myself acting the same way.*

At least he would be out of the way of my mom. We talked about all the things to do and see on Oahu. They were already excited about spending a week to explore Maui later in the summer with my younger sister when she visited from Boston. One of my brothers planned to fly out for a week with his girlfriend and stay in a hotel at Waikiki.

On the curbside at the airport, my parents announced they would re-arrange the furniture in the apartment as soon as they got back. "And you can't stop us." *Fair enough.* I gave my dad the car keys and waved goodbye as they headed toward the apartment in Manoa, near the University of Hawaii campus.

Well before my parents got to Honolulu, I found the US State Department Travel advisory on Nepal. Here was a long report which spoke in stark terms about the civil war. "Travel via road in areas outside of the Kathmandu valley is still dangerous and should be avoided." Now that the Maoists were part of the government, the US State Department regards the Nepali Government as condoning terrorism. I emailed a copy of the Travel Advisory to my relatives.

My younger daughter called in tears and implored me not to go. She cried as she reminded me of a long-ago promise to hike the Appalachian Trail with her when she graduated college. "If you die in Nepal now, you will not be much of a hiking buddy next year."

My younger sister also called and told me I was crazy. "You should believe the government when they give those warnings." A friend in Boston had a different perspective "So they think the Nepalis are terrorists? I bet if you asked the Maoists, they would say the exact same thing about the US government."

My older daughter, Julie, said, "Do you remember when we went to Disney World and the unofficial guide called it the Disney Bubble? That's what this is. You will be out from under the usual set of things we take for granted. That's what you have always wanted." She was referring to the way the theme parks package and filter a vacation experience. This also happens in the Caribbean, where any given resort has boundaries marked with barbed wire and patrolled by armed guards. If you walk out the gate used by the servants you can get to the hamlet just a mile away where the locals live, and things are not nearly so shiny and new. *These places are still beautiful – just in a different way.*

When she was high school, Julie had spent a year as an AFS exchange student in Brasil. She reflected on that adventure and said, "Go, but remember, once you have been that far out of the bubble, it's hard to get back in. Don't say I didn't warn you."

She was right – I was determined to go as far out of the bubble as I could get, for as long as possible.

"And one last thing, Dad. Don't go calling it the 'Third World' – that's considered to be insensitive. Call it something else – maybe 'Lesser Developed Country' – instead. That way you are less likely to piss them off."

My friend Celeste, who is Buddhist, said, "This trip will be a transformative experience for you." I was not sure what she meant by that.

Somebody had told me to look into International Health Insurance, so I could get evacuated to Singapore if I needed medical care. It was sobering to learn that *my part of rural Nepal was not covered. Period.* If I were to get sick, there was no way "out," and I would have to get medical care from the people with whom I worked. In March I went to the University of Hawaii travel clinic and got my immunizations. I sat with the doctor as he leafed through the recommendations, looking at the distribution maps of the various diseases. *No, I did not expect to do any spelunking or river rafting, or to handle livestock. No, I would not be traveling to altitudes above ten thousand feet.* In the end we decided on a boosters against tetanus, typhoid and polio. I had already had a hepatitis vaccine and the Measles, Mumps and Rubella combination. Nepal does not have Yellow Fever.

"What about getting the shot for Japanese B encephalitis and rabies?" I asked.

The doctor looked in his manual and said, "No, too much danger of an allergic reaction. And if they are having an outbreak, you will know. Save it for then." Then he wrote out a prescription for a bottle of Doxycycline. Tansen is above the elevation cutoff for the malaria zone, but I expected to travel through the lower elevations where malaria is a possibility. Also some Cipro, the nuclear weapon of antibiotics, in case of traveler's diarrhea.

The doctor studied one particular paper and cleared his throat before he looked me in the eye over the top of his glasses. He said in a grave voice, "I need to tell you that the prostitutes of Nepal are rife with diseases such as HIV and hepatitis. The condoms there may not be reliable."

"Thanks, Doc. I will keep that in mind." *The health problems of Nepal are the whole point of the trip.* I already knew about the human trafficking situation. The World Health Organization says that the only countries in the whole world with worse overall health statistics are Iraq, Afghanistan, and The Sudan. *I am glad he didn't feel like lecturing me on all the possible dangers, or we would have been here a long, long time.* I tried to keep a straight face.

In April I asked the people at the Tansen Nursing School whether I could bring something they needed. They asked me to bring any American nursing textbooks that I could spare, especially in the areas of Pediatrics and Mental Health nursing. I wheeled a cart from office to office collecting donated textbooks from my colleagues at UH Manoa. In the end I brought seven boxes of textbooks with me. Some of these books were still in the plastic wrapping. At the airport they weighed three-hundred-and-fifty pounds.

In my wallet there were ten crisp American hundred-dollar bills, since I did not trust the ATMs in Nepal and I knew that there would be no ATMs in Tansen. The exchange rate was seventy rupees to the dollar, so when I turned the dollars into rupees I wound up with five-hundred-rupee notes, one-hundred-and-forty of them, forming a wad in my pocket an inch thick. *This is like being a cowboy who just finished a cattle drive.* Over the summer I could measure the remaining time by looking at the wad of bills as it slowly diminished like a snow pile melting in spring after a long winter. As I rode toward Tansen, wondering what was going to happen when I got there, I took comfort in the fact that I was riding on the NGO vehicle, with UMN clearly marked on the side in both English and Devanagari.

Photo facing page: Morning at Guest House number four, the apartment for which I was charged $60 per month. Taken early in the summer, before monsoon. 300 staff and volunteers lived within the hospital compound.

Hiring My Didi

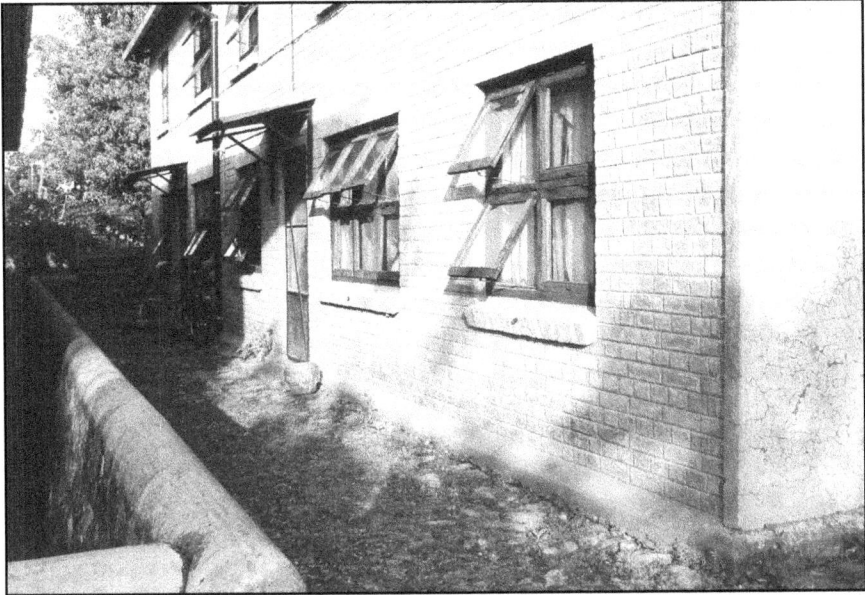

My initial view of the hospital was of the oldest part which was in the midst of an ambitious construction project. As I saw more I realized that it would not be so bad.

The day I arrived, I was warmly greeted by Ganesh, the Area Service Officer and manager of the Guest House. Ganesh is a local Nepali, tall and thin. He was friendly and cordial. He brought me to my apartment and gave me the key.

Ganesh told me to hire a *didi* from the list maintained by the hospital. The literal translation of *didi* is "older sister." My *didi* was named Bimla. She was a stout, cheerful woman, married with three kids. She was to be paid twenty-three rupees per hour, which worked out to about forty cents per hour. When she brought groceries over, Bimla always left an itemized bill.

The kitchen in my apartment was small but serviceable, with the same size refrigerator my daughter used at college. Every Monday, Bimla walked to the *Bajar* to buy groceries. This alone was worth the cost of having a *didi*. To do your own shopping would take too much time away from doing clinical work – first the walk to the *Bajar*, then learning where to buy each item, haggling over every price. For staples such as rice or flour, nothing came pre-packaged. Bimla would bring back a set of black plastic bags in to which the flour or lentils or rice had been poured.

She cooked for me as well. I hired her for eight hours a week, two four-hour shifts on Monday and Thursday. The plan was for her to bake cookies and make casseroles that could be eaten for several days. The first week she pre-cooked four quarts of rice for me to re-heat. People in Nepal eat a lot of rice, and she thought I would eat as much as the locals. On the table there was also a mountain of fruit. *Oh well, it's good for me.* I soon learned to enjoy the local fruit, especially the mangoes. There are mangoes in Hawaii, but in South Asia the mangoes are smaller and sweeter, with no oily or bitter aftertaste. We talked about the rice and she did not precook so much for me again.

To wash my clothes Bimla would put on rubber gloves, fill a plastic basin with soapy water, squat on the bathroom floor and scrub by hand. *One step removed from beating them on rocks.* The clothes would dry on a line outside. Later during monsoon we rigged up a clothesline inside the apartment.

Each building in the Guest House complex has its own barrels on the roof that are periodically refilled with a pump. The sink in the bathroom does not have a drain. It empties into a small bucket on the floor below. The water is saved and used to flush the toilet, which has no tank. Likewise, one stands in a big plastic tub when taking a shower. Later the shower water is recycled to flush the toilet.

The Asian-style toilet fixture is a porcelain trench, flush with the floor. The user straddles the trench and squats. To urinate in the trench is no problem, but like most westerners, I don't usually squat to defecate. Furthermore, the surrounding floor is always wet. There is no toilet paper. Use the left hand, then wash it carefully using a small bucket, after each trip. My first attempt to use one of these fixtures at the hospital was discouraging. *In Nepal, never touch a person or food with your left hand.* Happily the toilet in my apartment was a western-style throne. Within a day of arrival I personally went to the *Bajar* on a toilet paper purchasing mission. I was not quite ready to adopt every local custom.

Soon there was a knock on my door. I opened it to see a tall and pale woman, with circles under her eyes as if she had not slept well. She wore khaki pants and a casual button-down shirt. She introduced herself as Norma, one of the missionaries. She was here with her husband and two kids on a three-year tour. Today she was being neighborly, and taking a bit of time away from her duties as a pediatrician. As we walked to the hospital pharmacy to buy a bottle of iodine solution, she explained that she was from the Midwest, had trained in Wisconsin, and was board-certified in Pediatrics. Norma gave me a quick tour of the hospital.

My *didi* kept the iodine in the kitchen to soak vegetables and kill the germs on the outside of the vegetable. Norma told me never to drink even one mouthful of water from the tap, for fear of getting typhoid. *If I caught typhoid that would end the trip right there.*

Later in the summer, two Nepali coworkers came down with typhoid. It started with the usual classic headache and then got worse. They were too sick to get out of bed, let alone to travel. This made me even more determined to follow discipline as to the source of my drinking water. The idea that I might get sick and be forced to recuperate right here in rural Nepal was sobering. Typhoid can also be fatal. One night I lay awake thinking about this and reviewing in my mind the measures to avoid inadvertently drinking untreated water. I never opened my mouth when taking a shower. From then on I was careful to have a supply of bottled water, kept a small water bottle in the bathroom to rinse my mouth when I brushed my teeth.

The Christian Church in Tansen

People ask how I decided to do this, and how I got attached to UMN. There is a very simple answer. At the University I got an email asking for faculty who would agree to provide a lecture for a group of nursing students visiting from Japan. The topic was "Comparing the American and Japanese Health System" and it would pay two-hundred-and-fifty dollars. I enjoyed presenting the lecture so much I signed up to do it for the next few groups, and soon I had two-thousand dollars in an account. I went to the administrator in charge and asked how to get my money.

"Didn't you read the fine print of the contract you signed? You can't get paid that money in cash, my dear boy." He was looking at me over the rim of his eyeglasses. "It comes through a different route than usual, and you can only access it if you send a proposal to get reimbursed for an expense related to something related to international efforts of the University."

I was angry at first. I wanted my money. But the rules are the rules. So I decided to spend it on travel. *Two thousand dollars is enough to buy a round trip ticket to just about anywhere.* After all, I had just been to Singapore, and I was going to have three month's vacation in summer.

My first daydream was to spend the summer in Asia, so I did a web search. Nobody in India needs nurses. *Hey, type in the nearby countries, like Nepal.* That's how I found the site for United Missions to Nepal (UMN), an umbrella group of eight worldwide Christian churches. The website said they wanted surgeons, dentists, and the usual medical specialties. Scroll down, and the website also said they wanted volunteers to teach nursing. So, I sent a polite letter along with my qualifications. After a few emails it was done – now I would spend the summer with the Christian Missionaries. I was not some kind of "Official Missionary" myself. I had no goals and no expectations. *I was going to Nepal because it was cool.* When I worked in Nepal, I expected to do the same things I do at work in the US. Nobody really screened me regarding religious beliefs. I did not even have a *Bible* at the apartment – I was glad nobody asked.

Lately I go to the Catholic Church every Sunday, but this was not always the case. I lived in the State of Maine when my kids were little. My wife wanted me to accompany them to the United Methodist Church one Sunday morning in February. One Sunday I needed to stay home to work on correcting student assignments. I could listen to soothing music and enjoy looking at the stark winter landscape out the window. My wife packed up the kids and left in a huff. Over her shoulder she called me a mocking nickname, "Mister Spirituality."

Here in Tansen there was a full schedule of *Bible*-related activities. The daily medical staff meetings started with prayer. Wednesday evenings there was mid-week *Bible* study at one of the doctors' homes. Every Saturday morning in town, there was a Christian service in Nepali at a church near the *Bajar*, complete with a ten-piece praise band. Every other Saturday afternoon at the Guest House there was an English-language service run by the missionaries themselves. The hospital Chaplain Service consisted of two Nepali pastors, who made rounds on the wards every day and led a noontime prayer service in the hospital chapel.

There was only one other Catholic at the Hospital, so I decided to go the Hebron Christian Church every Saturday morning. It was a downhill walk from the hospital, and the first time I walked there, I was startled by two men on a motorcycle who rode up behind me without making a sound. They were coasting downhill to save gas. There was a pile of shoes outside the church door, just like in Hawaii. Old people sat in chairs in the back, but every one else sat cross-legged on the carpet. Men and boys sat together to the left of the aisle, women and children to the right. First there was an hour of music from the praise band. The repertoire consisted of old Nepali folk tunes with new Christian Lyrics. The congregation sang along. The sermon was in Nepali and lasted forty minutes. I looked over and saw that one of the American doctors was flipping through his *Bible*, meditating on his own. *He could not understand it any better than I could.* There was a point in the service where people prayed their personal prayers out loud – *it sounded like they were speaking in tongues. It wasn't English, that's for sure! Wow. Here I am with the Pentecostals.*

The leader of the band was the same man who served as the Hospital Chaplain, somebody who made rounds every day at the hospital. When I saw him next I spoke with him about joining the band. No problem. The next week I brought my trumpet. I packed it for the trip to Nepal because I knew it would open doors for me. I joined the praise band. Most of the members were in their twenties – a rock and roll drummer, two guitars and electric bass, a man about my age, playing the tambourine.

The small on-stage choir knew how to pump it up. The lead singer was a petite young woman who could really project her voice. If this had been western music, she would have been an operatic *coloratura*, or maybe Aretha Franklin. Her ear was tuned to the Indian scales and harmonies and she used a very high soaring register with ornamentation as if she was starring in a Bhangra video. The five others created electric energy when they sang backup. What surprised me was that some of the tunes were western hymns, but the band had the ability to overlay a harmonic structure to make the hymn sound as though it had been written in Kathmandu. *This blew my mind. Charlie Parker has nothing on these guys.*

I played along by ear. The tunes were not familiar to me, but I faked it okay and sat out when I could not get the key.

As the congregation sang the hymns, the sound was directed to the stage which seemed to make it louder. The time came for the personal prayers and the elevated stage provided a unique vantage point. I could look down on the colorful clothes and faces of the worshippers. During the part where the individual prayers were being offered, the hands were raised and formed a forest of arms. Faces were upturned, people craned their necks to the sky... eyes closed... men prayed loudly; some women with tears streaking down their faces as they murmured their heartfelt desires... in communion with God... and everyone swaying back and forth while the guitar played softly in the background.

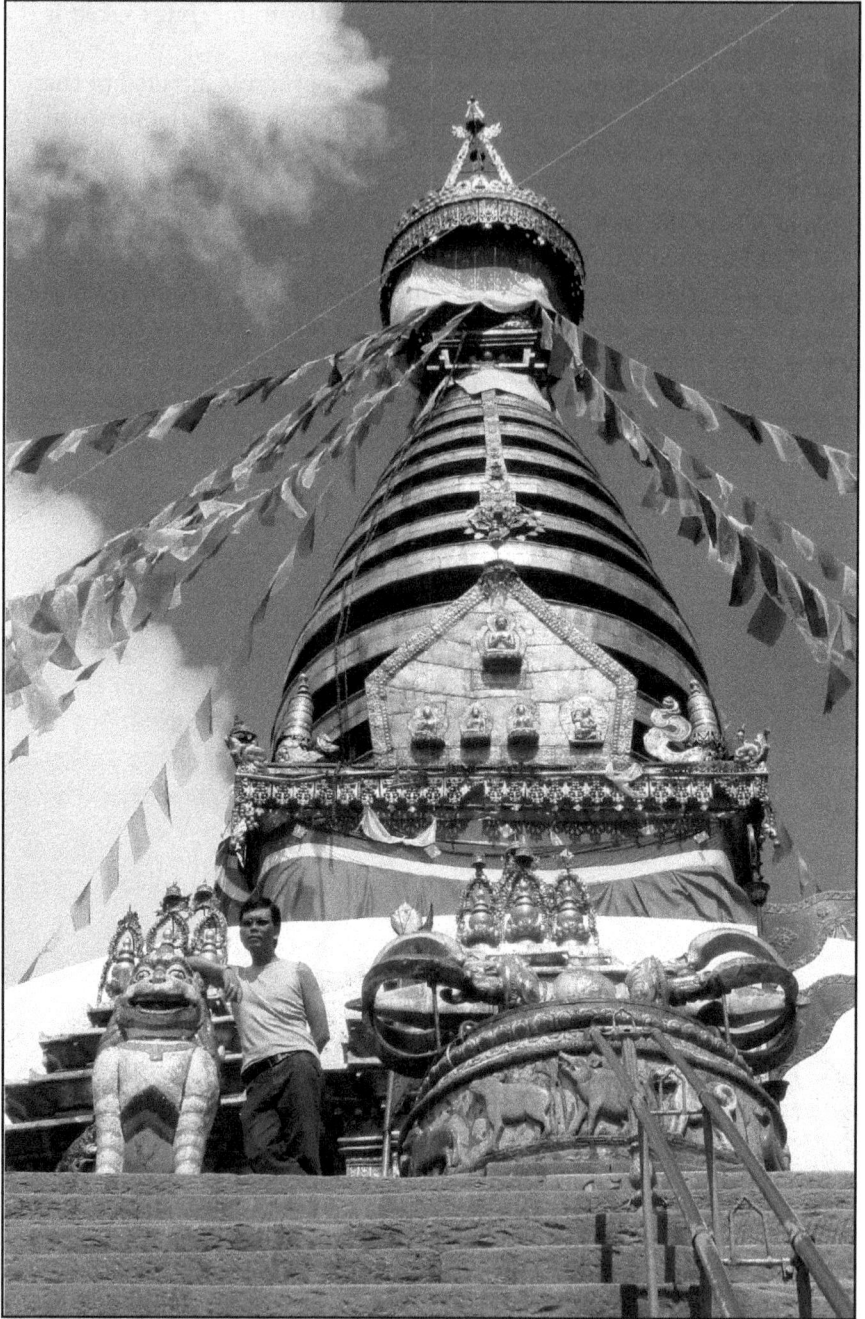

Swayambunath, which overlooks the Kathmandu Valley, is sacred to both Hindus and Buddhists. Pilgrims to Swayambu can take a two-miles-long Kora route which circumnavigates the entire hill upon which Swayambu stands.

Celeste

The year before I decided to go to Nepal, I taught an introductory course in nursing that dealt with issues of professionalism. Nurses need to study topics like how to develop habits of learning throughout life, and how to relate to people who are suffering. In Hawaii many of the students have Asian Buddhist backgrounds. They told me, "Joe, you are a Buddhist and you just don't know it." I was skeptical when they told me this, but at their urging we invited a Buddhist to come to class. There are two Tibetan *lamas* on Oahu and they live at a small Tibetan temple in a residential neighborhood. The older *lama*, who spoke better English, arrived wearing his saffron and yellow robes. He spoke eloquently about suffering and patience.

A few weeks later I attended the evening prayer service, known as *puja*, at the Kagyu Thegchen Ling temple. Here was a religious tradition of which I was ignorant. Most of the time there would be just a dozen or so people sitting on the pillows. They chanted in halting Tibetan. From a musician's point of view they did not have enough critical mass to get a good rhythm of Tibetan-style chanting going.

In October a famous Tibetan Rinpoche named Mindrolling Jetsun Khandro came to Honolulu to give teachings on Buddhist philosophy. I learned that a *Rinpoche* is a reincarnated master of Buddhist wisdom. The picture on the flyer showed a person with a shaved head, so I was surprised to learn that this *Rinpoche* was a woman. The retreat lasted Thursday evening through Sunday. I looked forward to the opportunity to hear a well-thought out scholarly discourse, so signed up for all four sessions. It was billed as a systematic overview of Tibetan Buddhism as described in the book, *Thirty-Seven Practices of a Boddhisattva*.

During each of these days the audience sat cross-legged on the floor, preparing for the arrival of the *Rinpoche* by meditating for an hour. Sometimes it would be silent, other times we would say *Om Mane Padme Hum* as many times as we could. Fifty people sitting on the floor, fingering prayer beads, saying the mantra at their own speed. For the retreat, the local Buddhists mustered up more than the usual number of attendees, and the room was full. When the *Rinpoche* arrived, there was a flurry of bowing and murmurs of *Namaste* while everyone settled in for the lecture.

My attention was riveted during the first two evenings of the retreat. The *Rinpoche* talked about patience and how to respond to anger. Anger destroys *karma*. Buddhists work to remove anger from their life, including getting away from angry people. This hit close to home, and I found myself thinking about the issues in my life from a new perspective. I had been married a long time to a beautiful woman from Boston, as Irish as could be, complete with red hair and freckles. We were now separated; for two years we talked of divorce. Early on, our relationship was a source of love and acceptance as we raised two daughters on an old rundown farm in Maine; but when the girls grew up and left the house we seemed to lose that sense of togetherness. We were strangers in a way. Our relationship became defined by anger all the time, anger that wore me down. That was how I ended up in Honolulu in the first place, officially separated.

There I was, dealing with issues of anger for years, and I needed to recoup my self-esteem. And now at this retreat I had a new way to look at my problems. *Anger destroys Karma.* The Buddhists said the way to get anger out of my life was to get the angry people out of my life. *And get the divorce.*

The morning of the third day, I bought the last copy of the *Thirty-Seven Practices of a Boddhisattva* book before the lecture started. I was flipping through the pages when somebody sat down beside me.

"Can I look at your book? You bought the last copy!" I looked up from my reading to see an Asian woman with long black hair braided down her back, smiling at me. Of course I had noticed her before – who wouldn't have? She had a beautiful smile and a way of giving you her full attention when she spoke. I had seen her sitting nearby during the sessions. She was dressed in black and I thought maybe she was in her late thirties. She was Asian, but somehow she was not as reserved as many Asian women in the room. That was why people seemed to gravitate around her. I thought she might have glanced over my way a few times. I thought about talking with her, but I was probably the only guy in the room who had ignored her. Maybe that's why she came over.

"Here." I handed it over and she started flipping through it. "You get it for five minutes free, after that I will have to charge you."

"I can't read that fast." She sounded like she was from the mainland; she did not have the soft music of the local Hawaiian accent.

"Are you from California?" I asked. *That was a guess.*

'How did you know? I am from San Francisco."

"Well, because I thought I may have remembered you from that time in North Beach. You know, back when you made a fool of yourself." She knitted her eyebrows together and seemed to catch herself for a bit.

Then I said, "I'm kidding, I haven't been to San Francisco in twenty-five years." With that she took a deep breath, and reached out to squeeze my bicep with both hands.

"O God, you had me going there for a bit!"

"I couldn't resist." We introduced ourselves. Her name was Celeste. Then I asked how she was enjoying the retreat.

"It's a new paradigm for me. I am particularly interested in the part about anger and how to develop patience." I was a bit surprised. *Paradigm. When was the last time I heard anybody use that word in a sentence in casual conversation?*

We talked for about ten minutes before the meditation started. Like me, she thought the part about patience was a key teaching. She said, "I'm working on anger every day, and this is so helpful." She smelled nice, but I could not make out the scent. She sat near me that morning, and I noticed that she could do the lotus position without the need to shift position. She kept her spine straight and I don't think she fidgeted once. As soon as the two-hour break for lunch started, she asked about borrowing the book. I agreed to lend it to her if I could get her contact information and phone number. She took the book and I watched her step out the door and find her sandals. As she slipped them on her feet I saw that her toenails were painted bright red. She disappeared down the street to her car.

She missed the afternoon session and did not come back for the last day. I looked for her. *Guess I will never see that book again.* At the end of the retreat I made a donation. For each person who donated ten dollars the *Rinpoche* would place a *kata*, a white scarf, around the neck as she gave a blessing. I made the donation and took the *kata* home to hang in my living room, as a reminder to develop patience.

I called Celeste that evening and she answered the phone. She apologized for leaving without telling me. She had to work, and could not afford the Sunday session. *She wasn't stealing the book or anything.* She loved Buddhism, especially the Tibetan kind, though she was raised Catholic. She attended *puja* every few weeks. Her favorite was *Tara Puja*, she said.

"That's on the Full Moon, and it's when we give offerings to Tara, the Goddess. I love how the Tibetans still believe in the Goddess, don't you?"

"Somehow I missed that part when the *Rinpoche* was here. What do you mean?"

"The Tibetans believe in the Goddess, that's what I mean. Her name is Tara. Also, when a woman meditates, a spirit called a *dankini* can come to inhabit her body."

As we spoke I learned that she had been in Hawaii a year. Celeste was from the Bay Area and had no family in Honolulu. She worked at a preschool and had a part-time job as a tutor on weekends. Later I learned that she was born in Asia and had been adopted by a family in California, which explained why she was so self-assured and outspoken compared to most Asian women in Hawaii. She was proud to say that she was from the SoMa neighborhood of San Francisco. In my mind, I scrolled through the neighborhoods of The City, finding no memory of SoMa from when I went to graduate school there. SoMa was evidently new since the dot com era. Celeste also told me she had lived in Bali once, and traveled through Asia, but not Tibet or Nepal. She enjoyed yoga and was a certified instructor. I told her about my job at the University.

Two weeks later I took a business trip to Singapore, a consulting trip on nursing continuing education that had been planned since June. I loved Singapore. I was eager to visit Asia again. I thought about teaching nursing in Singapore in summer 2007. I wanted to get a bit further out of the bubble of western society though, and Singapore was too tame, too westernized.

Things developed slowly with Celeste, but a couple of times I picked her up in my car and we went to dinner. Celeste was adamant that we were not "dating" – it was "hanging out." She knew I was getting divorced and I think that made her a bit cautious. She was a bit evasive and mysterious about her own situation. "Just looking for the right guy," she would say. My divorce was finalized that winter.

One day in mid-March the phone rang. I was surprised to hear Celeste's voice, because we had not spoken in a few weeks. This time she was in tears, with periods of silence interspersed by sobbing over the phone. I thought maybe somebody in her family had died. She was having trouble getting the words out. After a minute she was able to tell me she had gotten a bad performance evaluation at work. She started to tell me how hard working she was and how her boss acted like a jerk. I could hear her anger welling up. It turned into a tirade with threats of a lawsuit. She went on and on. After listening for about ten minutes, I thought, *God, calm down.* It was really the first time I had heard Celeste when she was so angry. *Now I see why you need to study Buddhism*, I thought to myself. I told her to bear with me and try a small visualization. *Logic will not help here. Time to take the Tantric path on this one.*

"Just close your eyes and picture your self planting a small bomb under her chair. You are somewhere else when it goes off, and nobody suspects you. She is blown to smithereens. Later it is announced that she was stealing from the milk money, and her reputation is disgraced forever." I gave the longest description with every embellishment I could think of, and drew it out for a few minutes. She chuckled at the fantastical details and said that it sounded about right.

"Now picture yourself coming to work the next day. Your new boss tells you to clean up the mess." At which point she laughed. I knew she hated cleaning. That seemed to break the ice and help her to re-frame the situation. "So you see, the bomb doesn't really solve anything even though you feel good for a bit. There will only be the next thing, after this." I then said, "Ask yourself the following question – is this the hill you want to die on?"

Later that week she sent me a card saying, "Thanks for helping me when I was not in my right mind, or my left mind for that matter." She managed to patch things up and decided not to change jobs. I learned later that she changed jobs every year or two.

After that we started seeing each other again. She sometimes would not return my call for a few days. On weekend mornings her voice was husky and she seemed irritable. She loved foreign films, and we could discuss the cartoons in The New Yorker since we both subscribed. I loved to talk with her, and I have to say that I loved her, period. She was a bright spot in my life during a time when things were changing for me.

One day we hiked Diamond Head, the extinct volcanic cone overlooking Waikiki which is an icon of Honolulu. It's only about seven hundred vertical feet, and soon we were in an unspoken contest to climb the hill. She got to the top first but I think she was surprised how I could keep up. Usually when I saw her she seemed to be wearing the same kind of clothes a bank teller would wear, along with manicured nails and tasteful lipstick. She usually wore Japanese-style platform slippers that added two inches to her height. If she had worn them on the Diamond Head hike I would have beaten her easily.

We ate at a Japanese seafood place the day I told her about my travel plans. I knew that Celeste once visited India with her college boyfriend, but did not know the details. "I was not used to traveling in places so hot and dirty. I volunteered at an orphanage and we went to see all these out-of-the-way temples. I spent most of my time arguing with my boyfriend and complaining about the heat and the bugs and the dirt and the crowds." I wondered what she was like in those days. There was still a lot about her I did not know. Despite her own experience with Asian travel, she was positive and upbeat when I told her about my plans. "This trip will be a transformative experience for you," she said. "Nepal is the place to learn about Buddhism, such a spiritual country. Maybe you can meditate at a *gompa* when you are there." All this time, she still had my Boddhisattva book. She kept promising to return it but I did not mind. As long as she still kept the book I had a pretense to call her.

The day before I left for Nepal, I excused myself from my parents and left them at my apartment where they were settling in. I drove down to Celeste's neighborhood, where she was waiting for me. She seemed happy to see me and we found a picnic table in Waikiki near the house where she rented a room. It was a sunny day in Hawaii which accentuated the green of the trees and the blue of the sky, and we settled down across from each other. The dark sunglasses hid her eyes, and her teeth seemed to sparkle in the bright sunlight as she smiled. She opened the bag of *sushi* takeout and gave me my chopsticks as we mixed the *wasabi* and soy. It was my going-away picnic. She doled out the *sushi* and explained each piece.

Celeste held the chopsticks, waving each piece of *sushi* in the air, then popping it into her mouth whole, as if she were swallowing a guppy. "It's the way you eat *sushi*." When the *wasabi* was too hot, she used one hand to cover her open mouth while she flapped the other hand in the air. She seemed to be looking at my reaction as if she was on stage acting out a part but desperate to know how the audience liked it. After the meal, Celeste rummaged through her purse and got out a small yellow silken cloth bag with a red purse string. She slid the little bag across the table and said "I can't give you a gift that costs a lot of money but these have their own value if you know how to use them. These are *Malla* beads. Use them to meditate in Nepal. This trip will be a transformative experience for you." Out spilled a set of small wooden prayer beads like chick peas. She showed me how to rub them between the palms to release the natural oils and a slight sweet spicy aroma. *Buddhist meditation beads.* We held hands across the table and I thanked her for this thoughtful gift. I carried the prayer beads in my pocket when I got on the plane for Nepal.

The Cardboard Box

After time on Surgical, Medical, Orthopedics, ER and OPD, I spent two days orienting to Pediatrics in mid-June. At that time I had no idea that I would later spend most of July there. In the mid-nineties I taught pediatric nursing for three years. It was while I was at my first teaching job, in Maine, but since then I have always thought of myself as a nurse who took care of adults.

While I was still orienting on Medical, I was approached by Samuel Luke, one of the pediatricians. "I heard that you brought the latest edition of Waley and Wong's pediatric book. Would you look in there to see what they have for a diabetic teaching plan for a school age child? We have an educator who can work with a Nepali girl with diabetes, but I want to make sure she is teaching the child the right things." I had seen him at church but this was really the first time we spoke about anything clinical. *How did he know what was in those boxes?* The boxes had gone straight to the nursing school. When I got to know him better, I learned that he was always thinking and planning. Samuel had a lot of projects cooking at any given time. My most vivid stories about Samuel deal with things he did in acute-care clinical situations, because that is where I saw him every day. But he also spent time meeting with people just to talk and plan and create a vision of what the hospital might do to better serve the people. His enthusiasm was infectious. He was also friends with the librarian at the nursing school.

I found the pages in the Pediatrics textbook and went to the administrator's office where the hospital kept the only photocopy machine. I took the pages to Samuel. The girl was eight. She had insulin-dependent diabetes, and the pediatricians thought that she would be dead by the time she was a teenager unless she could learn the new life skills of diabetes management. It would be a challenge. The girl lived in a rural area with no refrigeration or electricity. Her mother could not read. The girl would need to store her insulin, monitor her blood sugar, and give herself shots. In just one week, the girl experienced three episodes of hypoglycemia while still in the hospital. When the nurses were trying to teach her about her illness, she treated it like a game. Samuel arranged to get her a glucometer but the girl would not prick her own finger to get the drop of blood. The nurses were also new at using a glucometer. Samuel organized a tutorial for the nursing staff – a "toot." I thought this was a quaint term.

My first orientation day on Pediatrics was shortly thereafter. The census was fifty-three. Fifty in beds or cribs, and three on pallets in the hall. I started out the day observing doctors' rounds. Samuel was American, a board-certified pediatrician with training from a highly respected University in the Midwest. Samuel could speak Nepali very well. He always wore a *topi*, the cap worn by many Nepali men. I watched the reaction of people when they saw him in the *topi*. The Nepali patients seemed to relax and accept him completely. The *topi* also had the advantage of covering his bald spot.

I asked him about his last name. "Why do you not have an Asian-sounding last name?" Maybe this was too frank a question. "My family is descended from the Christians of Calcutta. Many years ago, that community decided to adopt their last names from books of the Bible. My dad was a urologist who moved to Ohio to practice, before I was born."

Normally Samuel led a team of interns and residents but this day there was only one resident to help examine each patient. The charge nurse of Pediatrics was there as well, and I was curious to see how they interacted. Samuel called her *Didi* and so did every one else. It was soon clear that they treated each other as partners and that the charge nurse was not shy about sharing her opinion, which Samuel took very seriously. I was pleased to see the teamwork and respect. Samuel began rounds in numerical order starting with bed one. He examined one patient at a time as the charge nurse recorded the verbal orders in a special notebook. In the first room was a young girl with a submandibular abscess. She came in with a reddened painful lump under her jaw the size of a ping pong ball and the lymph nodes below it were swollen. Her fever was now gone and the lump was not as big as it had been the day before. At the next bed we were looking at the abdominal x-ray of a child with typhoid, to see if there was "free air," an indication of bowel perforation. The next few patients were admitted with various upper respiratory tract infections.

After the sixth patient of the morning, Samuel was interrupted by one of the staff nurses. A baby in one of the isolettes in another room was doing poorly. We rushed to the room. An isolette is a crib with a plastic cover in which the air temperature can be controlled to prevent heat loss. Mission Hospital owned two and they were side-by-side in the same room near the nurse's station.

The baby was a preemie, only weighing four pounds, and had shown signs of respiratory difficulty when born at home. Here in the hospital her nostrils would flare as she breathed, and her ribs retracted as well, despite being on oxygen. She was also receiving nutrition *via* a tube. Now, she had stopped breathing. At first Samuel reached into the isolette and tried to assess her airway there. For me, I found myself looking up at the wall. *Where's the heart monitor?* It was a reflex to look up, because the monitor is usually mounted on the wall in hospitals in the US. I was jolted to remember that Mission Hospital did not have a monitor.

We found the orange plastic tool box that had the airway equipment in it, and spilled it out making a clatter. I started pawing through the pile, looking for the things we needed if we were going to get her breathing again. First, an ambu-bag to deliver small breaths – after all, she was a small patient. The next step would be to intubate – put a tube in to the trachea and use it to deliver oxygen – but this would require more than one person to accomplish and the isolette was against the wall. The room with the isolette was a cramped space in which to work. So Samuel picked up our tiny patient like you would hold a football, and carried her off to the treatment room. I started to follow but quickly ran back for the airway box, and threw the airway supplies back in the box. *We are going to need this.* I picked it up, and dropped an item or two as I hurried to catch up with Samuel trotting down the hall with the baby, the charge nurse, and the mom. We got to work as soon as we were through the door. Samuel laid the baby down, the charge nurse tinkering with the IV, while I opened the supplies onto the counter, spilling them like dice that have been rolled, looking for the laryngoscope and the right size tube.

We were in a room with a counter along one side and a long table with a plastic cover on a thin mattress. It was bare except for dressing supplies on the counter. Here, people could stand on both sides of the table and resuscitate the baby. The baby lay naked now, on the bare plastic of the table. I handed Samuel a number three tube and he confirmed that this was the size he wanted. Samuel positioned the laryngoscope and blade to insert the tube, and slid it into place. Anxiously, we listened for lung sounds – and heard them – which indicated that the tube was placed correctly.

When we hooked up the ambu-bag, we got immediate return of bright red foamy blood. *Dammit, this is not going well.* There was still no pulse. We resumed CPR, using two fingers to compress the tiny chest, but more blood appeared and we stopped. The baby had died. We stopped and silently looked at the baby. Its arms and legs were stretched out straight like a miniature grownup, not at all curved into the usual fetal position. The elapsed time was fifteen minutes.

When I write this I realize it sounds cold and clinical. Samuel was very methodical in the way he worked, remarkably composed, and I found that my old ways of working had kicked in so that we could focus on the task at hand. But the truth is that the mother was there with us every step of the way, and she was wringing her hands, flailing her arms and sobbing. This was the background as we kept working.

The day before, there were two babies in the isolettes. The newborn in the other isolette died at three in the morning, and the mother of the baby that just died had been there to watch the first one. In other words, the mother of this baby knew what was coming. She trailed along behind us when we ran to the treatment room, already crying. Now, the charge nurse stood by her side and rubbed her back, murmuring soft words.

Samuel soon matter-of-factly returned to rounds. An hour later we were dealing with another emergency – a six-year-old boy with meningitis who had been deteriorating for several days. He could not bend his neck, making a painful hunching gesture when we tested it for flexibility. He was now posturing and seizing uncontrollably. Right now, the IV was not working. Again we headed for the treatment room, with the mother trailing along behind. When we got to the door, Samuel abruptly turned to me, and commanded me to wait with the mother outside. This was a bit out of character for him, but I did as told and waited with the mother.

I got a quick glimpse into the room to see that the baby from an hour before was still lying on the treatment table under a small sheet. The mother of the first baby had left to get her husband, but he had not yet returned to retrieve the body of their dead infant child. Samuel and the charge nurse needed to figure out what do to about this while they focused on the patient who was still barely living. They did so with surprising rapidity.

Within fifteen seconds it was okay to come in. We worked to re-establish the IV on the seizing child with meningitis. *Where is the body of the infant?* I looked around. *It seemed to have vaporized into thin air.* As the child with meningitis seized, we could see the arm and leg on one side go limp, and we checked his eyes. One pupil had grown much larger than the other. The pressure had built up in his brain to the point where it was forcing the tissue to squeeze out of the base of his skull, a condition known as uncal herniation. He stopped seizing; and soon his pulse also stopped. He became limp. This one was not a candidate for CPR. There was silence in the room for a bit. I noticed that the boy' nose was snotty. I could hear my ears ringing.

And so it was – two deaths of children in two hours. As Samuel turned to this mother, she held the corner of her shawl to the lower half of her face and took deep breaths, groaning each time she exhaled, a cross between a sob and a sigh.

After a short period Samuel needed to return to rounds. As we left the room, he bent down to take a cardboard box that had been on the floor in the corner. It was the box which normally was used for soiled and discarded dressing supplies. His face was blank. He carried the box down the hall and gave it to one of the staff nurses. As he handed it to the nurse, I could see into the box. In it was the body of the preemie that had died, cushioned by the trash upon which it lay. He asked the nurse to take it out of the box, wrap it in a new cloth and get it ready for the parents. He then went back to work.

Samuel and I never spoke of this incident even once, but it was very vivid for me. *Mystery solved.* While I waited outside the treatment room with the mom, Samuel and the charge nurse placed the body of the first infant, into the box which contained the trash, the only place to conceal it from view. *Not very dignified. But what other choices were there in that moment,* I wondered. *None.* Here on the Pediatric Ward was where the rubber hit the road at Mission Hospital.

At noon, Samuel examined the six-year-old victim of a hit-and-run traffic accident the day before who was admitted with major scalp lacerations and blood in the ear canal. The neurological exams were good and the child was alert. The scalp had been sutured, and the child needed an ear exam. Samuel helped the father pick him up, and led the way out the door and down the ramp, to a musty corner of the hospital near the Medical Ward. We stopped as he got out a key and unlocked the door while the child whimpered quietly. The door opened to a brightly lit room which was cleaner than I expected given the dinginess of the corridor outside. Inside, was the endoscopy suite with a half-dozen endoscopes in suitcases, neatly stacked on shelves. Much to my surprise, there was also a surgical microscope, on a large arm with several joints such as a dentist might use to mount a dentist's drill. Samuel lay the child down on the endoscopy stretcher. He washed his hands, then whisked off a plastic cover of the microscope and found the switch, clicking it to brightly illuminate the child. He gently examined the child's eardrums, the good side first. He leaned back to let the father have a look. The drum on the injured side was intact and there was no blood behind the eardrum. After explaining what he was going to do, he delicately used a small probe to clear the scab from the ear canal. The child's hearing would be fine. Samuel looked at me and said he was Tansen's one-man Ear, Nose and Throat clinic. The microscope was the gift of a Swedish hospital, brought by a missionary a year or two earlier. Mission Hospital got a lot of stuff that way. The microscope was being put to good use.

As I left that day, I told Samuel I thought he needed a bigger entourage. He said he usually did have more residents to help with the daily work, but some were in Kathmandu taking an exam.

The next day I returned to Pediatrics. This time the pediatrician was the other American, Norma. She greeted me warmly and asked if I was wearing track shoes. Ward rounds started on the medical side, as usual and we worked our way through the first twelve patients. Norma always seemed so serious compared to Samuel. She seemed to be deep in thought at times, calling up the encyclopedic knowledge she stored somewhere deep in her head.

Communicable diseases seemed to be the theme of the day. The first two patients were toddlers with a diagnosis of A.G.E., which stands for "Acute Gastro Enteritis." They each came to the hospital with diarrhea severe enough to be life-threatening. The treatment consisted of oral rehydration therapy with *"Jeevan Jal,"* intravenous fluids, and Cipro. Each had responded overnight, each was producing an adequate amount of urine. The sunken eyes, a telltale sign of dehydration, had returned to normal.

"These children may go home later today. We have to make sure the report of the stool sample analysis comes back, to rule out typhoid or cholera," Norma said.

The next boy was about three-years old. His diagnosis was Pertussis. *Whooping Cough. Cool. I want to hear the "whoop."* I could barely contain my curiosity and eagerness to hear the characteristic whooping sound. Somewhere along the way in my career, I studied videos on childhood diseases which included the sound of whooping cough, but I had never heard the whoop in real life. In the US, you can go for an entire career and never hear the whoop. When you finally do, it is like being in the wild and hearing the call of a rare species of endangered bird. Norma could see my excitement and quietly explained that although Mission Hospital admitted a few such persons a year, this particular boy no longer had the cough, because he had coughed so much he now had laryngitis. With a smile she chided me for being disappointed. *Next time.* Whooping cough has a long recuperative period and can be fatal. This boy was on the mend, though it would take some time.

Sitting on the edge of the next bed waiting for us was a shirtless ten-year-old girl with Asian features and long black hair in a braid. She had been admitted with shortness of breath and was found on X-Ray to have severe cavitation of both lungs – probably tuberculosis. Her left lung was nearly obliterated. The girl was now breathing better. She was in a six-bed ward with other children who had breathing problems. She was thin with a protuberant abdomen and prominent ribs.

This girl was remarkably cooperative and unemotional while being examined. We needed to get a sample of the material that was clogging up her lung, but she was not able to cough any up for us, so Norma decided to do a needle aspiration.

"The biggest mistake people make with needle aspirations is to use a needle that is too small. This is thick material like mozzarella cheese, so we need the biggest needle we can fit between the ribs."

We walked hand-in-hand with the child to the treatment room and the girl dutifully climbed up, sitting on the edge of the table. Norma held the X-Ray up to the window so the light shone through, and counted the number of ribs down from the clavicle. Then she put the X-Ray aside, turned and smiled at the girl while she guided her fingers to count the same number of ribs, like playing "itsy-bitsy spider" until she got to the rib which correlated to the one she had found on the film. There she drew a small dot with a ball point pen. As the child looked at the mark, Norma assembled a small sterile field which included a number twelve needle on a syringe. This looked huge to me. Norma gave some local anesthesia and the girl did not even flinch. Next, Norma inserted the needle and tried to suck something out through it. Even with this needle size the material in the girl's lungs was too cheesy and sticky to retrieve a sample. I was worried that we would cause a pneumothorax, and collapse the lung if we punctured it by accident. Norma explained that the cavitation was so severe that the needle was well away from any functioning part of the lung. We put a Band-Aid over the site and went on to the next patient. The patient came along and got back on her bed.

The next boy also had TB; this was the miliary kind. The X-Ray of the lung was fine but there were little shiny dots like kernels of rice throughout his abdomen which gave it the name. He probably contracted this form of TB by eating something with the *bacillus* as opposed to breathing it into his lungs.

Later that day I also met Ramesh, a young boy who was all skin and bones when he arrived. He lived with his grandfather as his parents had died somehow. The grandfather was not exactly sure how old Ramesh was. Ramesh had complained of leg pain and was unable to walk. The X-Ray of his shin showed that all the marrow of his bone had been replaced by TB *bacilli*. The orthopedic surgeons wanted to drain this stuff from the bone, so they drilled a series of holes in the front of his shin. He now sported an area on his leg where about six inches of shin bone was exposed like ivory. The nurses would change the dressing on it twice a day. Ramesh was on a diet supplement now, and his weight was getting back to where it should be, or at least we thought so. Since we did not really know how old he was, we still were unsure as to whether he was now within the usual weight for his age. They also did not know whether he would keep the leg. When we did his dressing he would watch and turn it this way and that, wiggling his toes.

In yet another bed, there was a child with spinal TB. The patients at Mission Hospital presented with more manifestations of TB than I had ever dreamed to be possible. There were also a few children with Upper Respiratory Infection and some in whom it was necessary to rule out meningitis. For now it seemed as though everyone was improving. The second day on Pediatrics was much calmer than the first day had been. This was a relief.

Norma examined a thin little boy with intestinal worms. There were four main categories of worms in our area and he had some of each.

"A veritable Noah's Ark of worms," Norma said. The boy was underweight for his age, and also pale due to anemia. "When a person has hookworm, each worm creates a small ulcer on the inside of the intestine where it attaches, and these children are constantly losing blood into their stool."

We were collecting stool specimens; the container for these was unique – little clay pots, smaller than a shot glass, made at a local pottery shop with the texture of red brick. I took one as a souvenir.

I asked Doctor Norma about my immunizations. I got most of the shots before I came, but my doctor in Honolulu had told me I did not need Japanese B encephalitis because I would only need it if there was an outbreak. She said, "You should have gotten it. The turnaround time on the lab test for Japanese encephalitis here is so slow that we never know we are having an outbreak until weeks after it is over."

That afternoon as I walked along the gravel road between the hospital and the *Bajar*, I saw a blue tractor go past, pulling a trailer loaded with gravel. There seemed to be a lot of blue tractors in Tansen, and then I wondered, maybe there was only one tractor, a blue one, and it went back and forth continually, creating the illusion of more traffic than there really was. It made me consider how many private vehicles there were in Tansen, not many, and it seemed like the few cars in town were always chock full of people when they drove by. They went back and forth too, though most people walked everywhere, just like I was doing. I didn't really miss not having a car. It felt good to walk, and I recalled that somebody said hiking was the national pastime of Nepal.

On Flat Street at the *Bajar* there were three adjacent shops that specialized in *Palpali Dhaka* cloth and I picked the first one, which seemed to have brighter designs. You could buy a bolt of *dhaka*, or just a few meters, and take it to a tailor who would make clothes for you. And there were piles of *topis*, little caps, folded neatly and sorted according to size. This is what I wanted. My head is big and the shopkeeper shook his head at the way the first *topi* fit, but he rummaged around for a bag of large ones and I eventually bought a nice *topi* for one hundred fifty rupees. There were little Bo tree leaves in the design, representing the same kind of tree under which Buddha sat to achieve enlightenment. The colors included green, yellow, red, and blue over a white background.

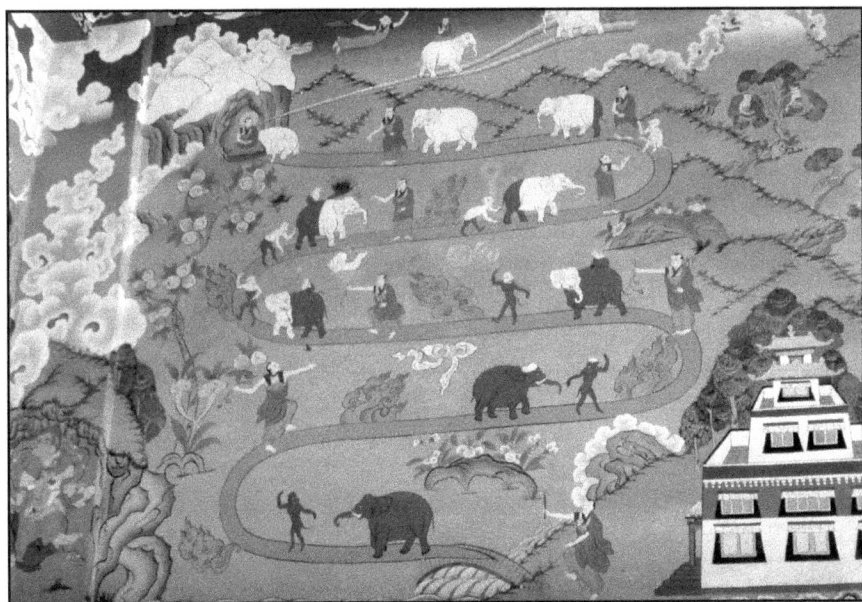

Kopan Monastery near Boudha. This mural depicts stages on the Path to Enlightenment. The elephant in the mural is transformed along the way.

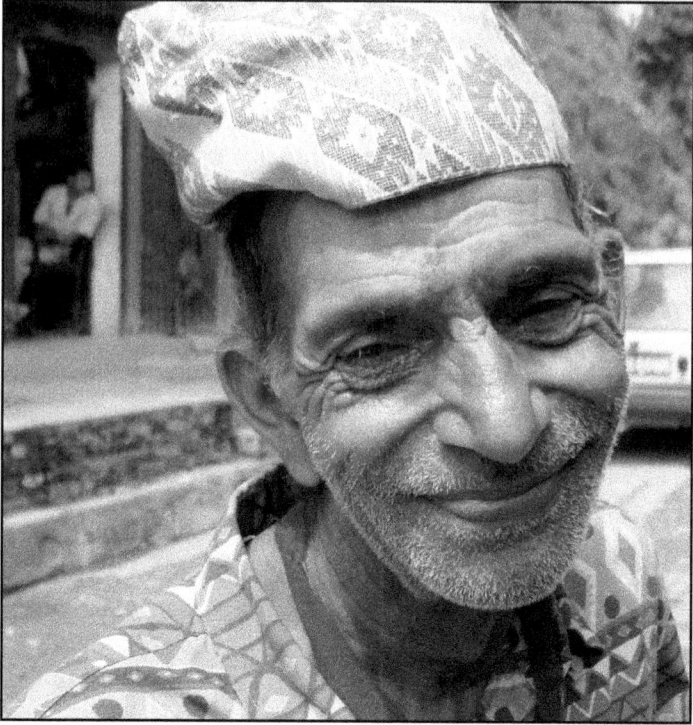

One of the locals wearing his topi at a jaunty angle on the day of a family party. A younger man would have worn it in a more formal fashion.

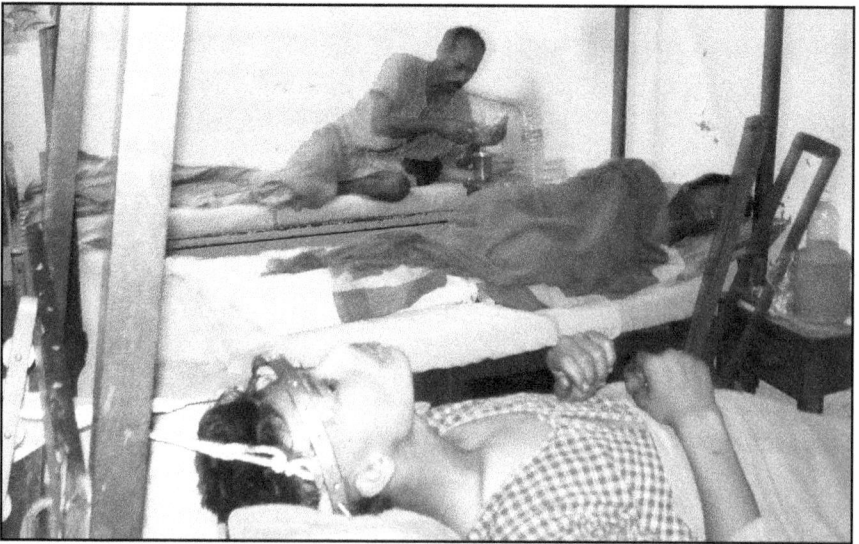

Men's ward, Surgical. Patient with neck injury on Halo traction in foreground. There were eleven beds in this room

Surgical Ward

After three weeks of orientation to the different service areas at Mission Hospital I reported to the adult Surgical Ward, to spend the last two weeks of June covering faculty vacations and supervising students in clinical practice.

Before I left the apartment I put the *topi* on my head and looked at myself in the bathroom mirror. *Well, this will get their attention. I wonder how it will go over. Will they laugh? Will they think I am being pushy? I won't know unless I do it.* I felt self-conscious as I took the short walk a hundred yards to the Surgical Ward. Outside my apartment door the crows had gotten into the garbage again. I heard them caw and thought they were laughing at me. The first person I saw was one of the *Chowkidars*, who smiled broadly. *Maybe this will work.*

A half dozen nurses were getting ready for the day, waiting for report when I appeared in the door. They all covered their mouths with their hands as they giggled and one of the younger ones said, "Sir, you are looking so handsome today!"

Over the course of the day, hospital staff went out of their way to come over and fuss over my *topi* and congratulate me for the design of *dhaka* cloth I had chosen. One of the Nepali doctors on the Surgical team took the *topi* off my head, refolded it to emphasize the crease, and ceremoniously placed it back saying I must always wear it so the rim was at *just* that angle. Not tipped forward, not tipped backward. Exactly horizontal. About five minutes later, one of the men from the ER came by and repeated the exact same process, taking theatrical pains to adjust it for me *just so*.

When the Medical team came by, another young doctor took me aside in a conspiratorial way and said, "On you, this *topi* is looking beautiful. But, if you really want a Nepali wife you will need to shave your mustache." We both guffawed as he slapped me on the back.

When it was time for *dal-bhaat*, the cooks at the canteen were wearing blue denim aprons and sitting out in the sun while they peeled huge bowls of potatoes and carrots. They also smiled. "You will be a real Nepali now!" From that day on, I always wore the *topi*. Over the summer I bought several more. My favorite was the one with the little Nepali flags in the design.

But this was the day to get down to serious business and actually do the job of supervising students. As in Hawaii, the activities of the day do not simply unfold. The students come with a list of tasks they have already performed; and there is a list of tasks and course objectives to be met. To a large degree my group was already self-directed; each one knew the general routine without being told. The incidental things that happen – patients to be admitted, post-op patients, and emergencies – are superimposed on this. So the challenge was to be well informed about each patient. I was in the habit of getting there an hour early to go over the list of patients, reading each chart in English before report started. Then I had to choose which ones to assign to each student for the day. I knew that if I wanted to have an easy day, I could assign patients who were not so sick. However, I always want to get into the thick of things, and in the US I was never afraid to assign patients who would need a lot of care from the student assigned to them. In Tansen I assigned a student to just about every patient on the ward. And since I was their teacher I could freelance around the ward offering my opinion with a large number of patients, more patients than if I was simply working as a staff nurse. I did not know how to do some of the simple clerical tasks, but the staff nurses were there as backup and knew how to do things like ordering meds or lab tests. To be there as a teacher was a good fit for me, an ideal role for an American nurse to work in a Nepali hospital.

The Surgical Ward has about forty beds and is located right outside the door to the Operating Theater. The Critical Ward holds five patients and is next to the nurses' station. As on Medical, the name does not mean that it had any extra monitoring equipment. On the other side of the nurses' station there are two, eleven-bed open wards where the beds are right next to each other, one for men and one for women. These are referred to as "Nightingale-style" wards, after a design popularized by Florence Nightingale in the nineteenth century – a big open room in which everyone can see everyone else, one bathroom for each ward, Asian style. This is a sharp contrast to the usual two-to-a-room of an American hospital. Early in my nursing career I worked in the Dowling Building of the old Boston City Hospital, which operated the last of the Nightingale-style wards of any hospital in New England. Because of that, I felt strangely at home as if stepping back in time. *Oh, to be young again!* I was twenty-two-years old in those days.

There are also some two-bed and four-bed rooms, and the usual spaces for pallets along the corridor. I was now accustomed to the idea that we would get overflow. Here at least, the corridor was a bit wider than the other wards and there was less through traffic.

On Surgical, I met my first patient with Kala-Azar, also known as visceral leishmaniasis. It is a communicable disease, but not catchy. A friend in the US military once told me the nick name for *leishmaniasis* was *"face-eating disease."* It was easy to see that this patient had the remnants of a now-healing rash on the lower half of his face. He lived in the Terai, where the sand flea transmits *Kala-Azar*. His spleen was the size of a watermelon, sagging his belly off to one side. He was stable now that he received four units of blood. He was getting a drug named "sfibonide", or "S.A.G.," which I had never used in the US. The active ingredient is antimony, a heavy metal.

In a nearby bed was a man with abdominal tuberculosis and ascites, a collection of fluid in the abdomen. He looked pregnant and his bellybutton was sticking out. He was in liver failure caused by a reaction to isoniazid (INH), an anti-tuberculosis drug.

In the next bed there was a trauma victim who had a chest tube in place, to prevent his lung from collapsing. The tube was hooked up to just one bag, which at first glance looked like the kind of simple collection bag we used only for urinary catheters in the US. I looked at it closely and realized that it still provided a water seal, but I was surprised to see that they did not use three-bottle drainage. The right side of this man's face was swollen beyond recognition. He hardly asked for pain medication despite his injuries. He was cutting firewood when he lost his balance and bounced down a stony cliff, breaking five ribs along the way before he landed in some bushes. His wife sat by his side wearing a Magar outfit complete with shawl though it was ninety-five degrees.

In the Gynae Ward, a woman with her arm in a sling displayed a huge welt on her neck. She was riding on the back of a motorcycle with her child in her lap, when the scarf of her *kurtha surwal* caught in the wheel, jerking her off the seat. She broke her collarbone and some ribs with a small hemothorax and a concussion. The child went flying but was miraculously unharmed. Other patients had gallbladder disease, foot ulcers, post-partum fever, and the like. All eleven beds on the Gynae Ward were occupied.

As we move down the corridor to the two-bed rooms, there was a twenty-seven-year-old man with a history of alcoholism who had been admitted with pancreatitis. Lots of local people made their own *raksi*, potent homebrewed alcohol, and we often admitted patients that had been beaten during some drunken brawl. This young man drank too much. Despite his youth, he was reaping the consequences of alcoholism. During the day he developed shortness of breath and pallor. He sat upright laboring to breathe. We called the surgical team and they ordered more oxygen. His dyspnea progressed, and the doctor thought he was in full blown Adult Respiratory Distress Syndrome, a complication of pancreatitis with a high mortality rate, even in the US. He soon was unable to sit up any more. The next morning when I got there early, he was in the last stages of death.

In a case such as this, there seemed to always be a point where those of us who had studied or worked in the West would ask, "What would have the outcome been if this person had been in an American hospital?" In the US, people with severe pancreatitis have a mortality rate of thirty per cent. Here it was one hundred per cent. We did not have the sophisticated therapy to save him. His father sat on the low wooden stool at bedside and watched his son float off downstream. The doctors checked in periodically and the nursing student gave morphine overnight. By morning, ten men stood silently by the father. When the patient stopped breathing, his father shouted at the doctors for about five minutes. After a short while the men matter-of-factly moved the body onto a stretcher using a three-man lift like a drill team. One man had tears running down his cheeks, and it was only then that I realized that the group of men had assembled specifically to conduct the Hindu rituals of death. There were no women among them. Later the men would use the same three-man lift to place the body onto the funeral pyre. We continued with our other work for the day.

I met my first "neural leprosy" victim on Surgical, a sixty-year-old man with an infected foot. I was expecting to see a person with severe disfigurement, like a walking image from the *Bible*. Here I learned that this is more than one kind of leprosy, and his type was mainly characterized by nervous system impairment, including numbness of extremities and inability to close one's eyes. In his foot, was a crater about an inch across and deep enough to see the metatarsals at the bottom. The wound was neat, as if it had been drilled with a woodworking tool. It was painless. His face was waxy and his stare made him look threatening. Despite his ominous appearance, he turned out to be a sweet and gentle person. He was not on any anti-leprosy medications when he arrived. He was now going to be enrolled in the Leprosy Clinic. Leprosy is not covered very well in textbooks from the US. When I asked around, a faculty member from the Nursing School gave me her copy of *Common Medical Problems in the Tropics*, by CR Schull. She was going to throw it away because it was moth eaten. I took it home and it became my bedside reference. I devoured it more thoroughly than the moths had.

Another day on Surgical, a man my own age was admitted to the eleven-bed ward with abdominal pain. The ER doctor took an EKG and also some X-rays, looking for an air-fluid level that would have indicated a perforated intestine, but this did not appear on the X-ray. The patient produced his old medical records in a wax-paper envelope; and the history indicated a prior diagnosis of Buerger's disease, an abnormality of blood clotting. He was first given to the surgical team, and they proceeded through a list of "rule outs." In layman's terms, this meant they did not know for sure what it *was*, but they would make a diagnosis after deciding what it was *not*. His right leg had previously been amputated above the knee. It was curious to note that he had no body hair, not even any pubic hair. There was a *janai* around his waist, the string to indicate that he was a devout upper caste Brahmin. He had a "*topi*" of scalp hair - indicating that about six weeks previously, his hair had been cut in a certain way as a sign of mourning. Most of the head is shaved except for a small topknot. Nobody ever got to ask him who might have died, probably his father.

Our Brahmin patient had intense abdominal pain accompanied by liquid diarrhea, foul smelling and the color of bile. During the first hour of the shift, two doctors of the surgical team were excused from ward rounds so they could focus on his diagnosis. They crowded around him and decided that he was not a candidate for surgery. The medical team was then called. They had their own list of "rule outs," starting with a repeat EKG which was normal except for tachycardia. Al, the medical student from the UK, was there and I told him that I could not recall anything like this patient - if the doctors could not figure out what was wrong I did not think I could.

I hovered a short distance away, watching the doctors asking questions while doing physical exam maneuvers to diagnose his problem. The nursing student I assigned to him was a first-year and I made sure she was helping with vital signs and keeping him comfortable. The man vomited, and the material was the exact color and consistency that his diarrhea had been. He sank back on the bed. From a distance, I could see his mouth twitch as if he was a fish out of water. He had stopped moving any air. I hurried over and asked the nursing student for her stethoscope. I could not hear a heartbeat. I looked at the medical student from the UK. "Al, can you hear a heart beat?"

Al was visibly galvanized by this question and grabbed the stethoscope while I felt for the man's carotid artery. No pulse either way. Al started CPR and we sent for the airway box. While the resident prepared to intubate, the man vomited again. I pulled the gloves out of my pocket and put them on, as we had to turn him on his side to clear out his mouth. He was limp like a sack of flour. The skin of his neck and upper torso turned blue in a particular pattern which we recognized as "cape cyanosis." His jugular veins were popping out, like twin snakes under the skin. The nurse quickly brought the portable suction, but it was not sucking up the vomit fast enough. The bed was a mess, and as we knelt to do CPR we were getting his vomit on the knees of our pants. *I wonder what Celeste would think if she saw me now.* The resident called a halt. We looked at the patient, his unmoving eyes staring up at the ceiling, no longer twitching, and I still wondered what his medical problem was – maybe a mesenteric thrombosis. Al and I looked at each other and shook our heads ever so slightly with the eye contact. He had a quizzical look.

"Don't ask me what just happened, " I told him. "I don't know what this whole episode was about." *Hell, if I had even a clue as to what was wrong with the guy, I would have told them.*

It was then that I noticed the rest of the patients on the ward; suddenly I was conscious of their presence. The whole affair was conducted in public from the time of admission early that morning. All the other patients saw the groups of doctors, the activity, the discussions, the orders, and finally the CPR. We had not closed the drapes to create the illusion of privacy, but even if we had, it would not have shielded the other patients from this scene.

For the rest of the day, I continued my usual pattern of going from room to room to check in on the students, as if I was doing laps on a treadmill. Every time I entered the eleven-bed men's ward I would say *Namaste* to no one in particular. If a patient was watching, they might return the gesture, silently. That day, when I entered the ward again, they added the response *Hajur*, which meant "Sir." This Nepali word conveyed a tone of respect such as you would give to an elder of your village or a person of higher caste.

Later that day somebody told us that it was clear enough to see the Himalayas. Above the hospital and the shantytown there was a concrete stairway with five hundred steps leading to the top of Shree Nagar hill. I climbed up with my camera. It was late afternoon, and the distant mountains shimmered with red alpenglow above a wreath of clouds. It was hard to believe the peaks were more than sixty miles away. Annapurna was surprisingly tall even from that distance. I took pictures. Once the monsoon started, the Himalayas would be clouded in. I think I only saw the mountains one other time.

That evening I ate in my apartment, then headed up to the Guest House for some after dinner conversation with the medical students. They enjoyed their meat loaf and potatoes along with a salad of sliced cucumbers and tomatoes. Padma, the other medical student from the UK, was there, deftly using the spoon to pund her teabag against the saucer, over and over, in various positions. She was fresh from a day on the Maternity Ward learning how to check a woman's cervix for effacement and dilation. Padma was enthusiastic about the new assessment skill she was acquiring.

For the uninitiated, a woman's cervix is a narrow spot in the birth canal, which must open for the baby to be born. You can not see it; the only way to measure the degree of openness is to feel it with your fingers. The examiner will place a sterile glove on one hand, then slather it with a liberal amount of sterile lubricant. Two fingers are placed gently and deeply in the place where the baby will later emerge, and the cervix is prodded and examined. The information obtained this way is used to predict the progress of labor. The skill of cervical examination is honed with guidance and practice. Padma had done it a dozen times that day. She was "getting it" and applying her new knowledge. We all enjoyed seeing her enthusiasm.

Al and I had a short discussion about our *Brahmin* patient. He had not noticed the man's *janai* and did not know the significance of the *topi*. Neither of us could devise any new explanation for the man's demise. We agreed that the vomit and the stool were disgusting.

"Ever heard of the 'fecal veneer?' " I asked. Padma chortled, suppressing a laugh.

"Enlighten me."

"The idea is, there is a thin film of fecal contamination on everything humans touch. It's a public health concept. Despite the emphasis on not touching anybody's left hand, I think the fecal veneer of Nepal is thicker than some other places. Possibly explains why people here don't touch each other very much."

"Not a reassuring thought. Today we broke through to the other side if you ask me."

"Did you get the hepatitis shot before you came?"

"Of course. I wonder what else we were exposed to with that little escapade."

Dessert was sliced mangoes and bananas mixed together. I spooned some into a dish for myself even though I had not signed up for supper. I had washed my hands before sitting down at the table, but they still felt dirty and I was conscious of the way the spoon felt on my fingers. I wished there was some whipped cream to top it off.

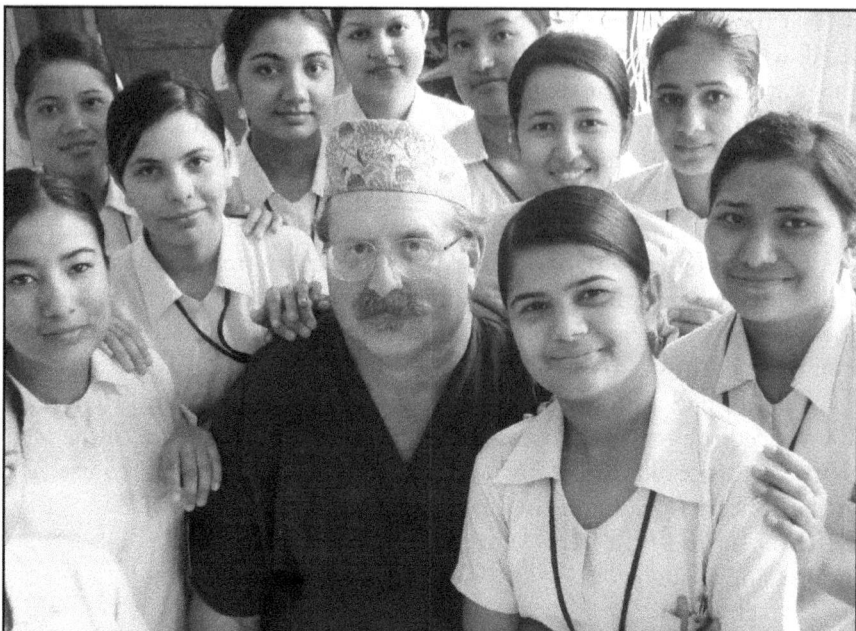

With a group of students from Tansen Nursing School. Note the topi. Students always wore the traditional nurse's cap and each carried the exact same items in their pocket.

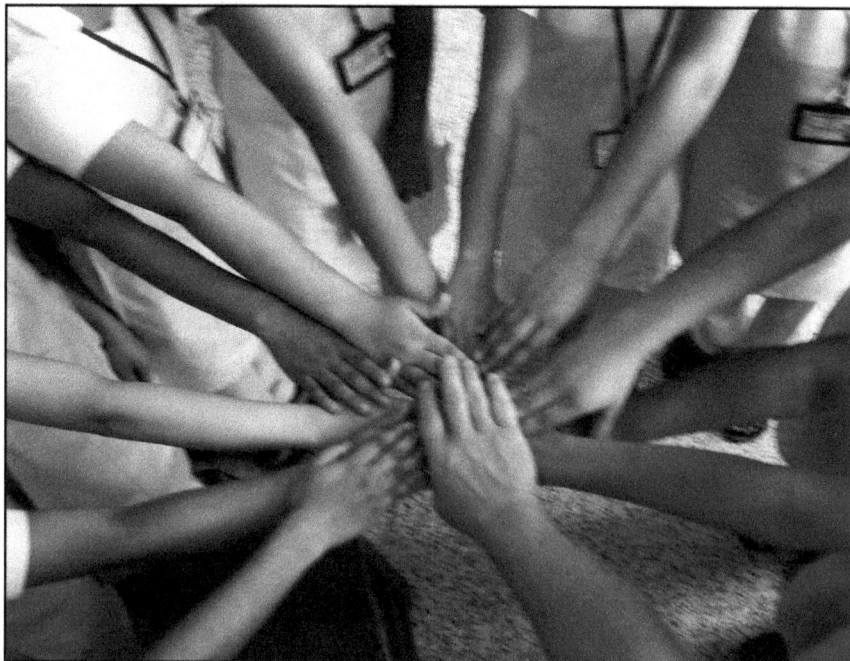

The Huddle. I use this with students both at UH and TNS.

Working With Beginner Nursing Students

On Surgical, one of the two groups of nursing students was nearing the end of their first year which meant that their average age was short of seventeen. At the University of Hawaii, the comparable students would be about twenty-years old. I had never worked with such young nursing students before. There were also some third year students on the ward and they were almost nineteen. When the students were from two skill levels, it was customary to have two faculty members on each ward. I shared this faculty posting with Arupa, one of the experienced teachers. She was about my age. For now I was covering the vacation of Arupa's usual partner, Ruth. When Ruth returned from her trip home to Korea, I would cover Arupa's vacation.

The first day began when the students at the nurse's station jumped to attention as I walked through the door, with bowing heads and a chorus of, *Namaste Sar*! I looked at them and asked the group to join me in the storeroom near the nurse's station. I told them I did not bite, and explained how we would "huddle" during the day. Like a basketball team on a time-out, I extended my right hand toward the center of the circle, and made a trembling motion with it, signaling that they were to do the same. They giggled, but first one, then more, stood closer and extended their hand, on top of mine. There were a few sheepish expressions, and they were tentative at first, but soon they all joined in, hands outstretched. I told them that whenever I stood in one place with my hand like that, it was a nonverbal signal for them to come over to listen. We would periodically use a short huddle during the day to coach them on various things that would come up. This was new, and they giggled and smiled when we did it. The group caught on quickly when we needed to confer with each other. From then on it we did it every day.

Every nursing faculty member needs to come to grips with the idea of working with beginners. I was not always patient enough for this assignment. Long before I studied Buddha, I already had one easy trick that kept me patient and humble. My daughters were now in their twenties but I could easily think back to their teenage years when they took Driver's Education. I could vividly recall the first few times sitting in the passenger seat while Julie, and then Amy, got behind the wheel. Getting a driver's license is commonly seen as a rite of passage for a new driver, but it is also a rite of passage for the parents.

A person who teaches nursing will often stand on one side of the bed to watch a beginner student do a skill on an actual patient such as giving a shot or adjusting a medical device, prepared to intervene if things don't go well. No matter how many times the student has practiced on a manikin, the student can be anxious. If the procedure has many steps, the anxiety gets in the way of proper technique. The teacher needs to be patient and calm in this situation. For me I could always recognize the change in my own tone of voice that indicated impatience. When that happened, I would close my eyes for a second and say to myself, *What if that girl across from me was Julie or Amy back at that age, two girls I love, and I was trying to see that they "got it?"* Usually this simple image was enough to help me regain perspective and proceed. I could find the language to break the ice and help the student succeed, without using sarcasm or belittling them.

The first year students were working on simple tasks such as vital signs and dressing changes. Each one carried a checklist of skills to complete, about fifty items. At the end of the week, the students brought their checklists to me for a signature to verify what they had done. For some reason they thought it was cool to get a signature from me, the American man. The checklist was in English, but I signed these using the Nepali script, which amused them. I would also use the Nepali to write short comments, such as *derai ramro!* which meant "very good!"

Lounging on a bed in a corner of the men's ward was a young man about sixteen. Until recently he had been a day laborer shoveling gravel. He had been standing too close to the blue tractor when it ran over his foot. The large rear wheel had made a fillet out of the front of his leg, scraping away the skin down to the bone. Right at the joint of the ankle, the place where a westerner would tie their shoelace, you could see the bone looking like the knuckle of a ham. The rest was raw meat. We were cleaning the wound and getting it ready for skin grafting. For his pain, he got two paracetamol - Tylenol - every now and then. The typical dressing we used for a large wound that was being cleaned and prepared for skin grafting was a "betadine wet to dry" dressing. He hopped around the unit on crutches and sometimes I would hop along side him and pretend to challenge him to a race. We might hop for ten feet and both laugh.

One day at ten in the morning we were working our way through the list of dressings to be changed in the eleven bed men's ward, and in walked the chief nurse for the entire hospital. Ambhika was a bright woman about fifty years of age, who wore a *tika* on her forehead to indicate she was Hindu. Mission Hospital had sent her to Vellore, India to get a Bachelor's degree from a Christian nursing college there. She was one of the "Sisters," meaning that she was fully qualified under the old Nightingale system of nursing education. Most nurses at Mission Hospital wore a western style uniform, but Ambhika was the only one to wear a pink sari under her lab coat, meticulously pleated. As she joined me watching the student do a wet-to-dry dressing, she wanted my opinion about the system for dressing changes at the hospital. Should they be using betadine on the wounds? She seemed relieved when I told her I thought they had a fine way of doing it.

Evidently an American nurse from the east coast had visited Mission Hospital the previous year and she was critical of the way the Mission Hospital nurses did their dressings. The last American had been trying to get them to use alginate dressings and wound vacs, now being used in the US. There was no way Mission Hospital could ever afford these new systems, and Ambhika was defensive about the standards of care used by the nurses. I could see her viewpoint, and I thought to myself this is not the way to elevate the standards. *Sure it would have been great if Mission Hospital could have better technology, but there needed to be a way to match it to the local reality.* I was working on the mechanical ventilation policy at this time and I made a mental note to keep Ambhika informed.

A week later, Ambhika came down with typhoid. She would be out of the picture for a month while she recuperated. The young man with the shin wound ultimately got his skin graft and was discharged. He was going to return in a few months for tendon surgery, but in the meantime he could gain strength at home. I saw him at the *Bajar* later in the summer without crutches. He was not able to move his ankle well, but otherwise okay. We hopped side-by-side down the street for a bit and shook hands.

Padma and the Tuscany of Nepal

There were two medical students whose time in Tansen roughly corresponded with mine, Al and Padma. Padma arrived after I had been there a month. When we first heard she was coming, the rumor went around that she was from Paris, and of course Al and I speculated about this at the dinner table while the orthopedic surgeon from Japan listened and chuckled – visions of dinner conversation with a woman who had a French accent. *God, what if she owned a beret? What if she could sing in French? Maybe she would wear Chanel Number Five.* .... How elegant! How wonderful!

In reality she was not French, did not own a *beret* and she spoke with an upper-class British accent. Her real name was Carol Ann, but everyone called her Padma. Her dad was Scottish and her mom was from Gujerat, a province of India. Padma grew up near London and was a second year medical student in the UK. She was the only party-of-one woman traveler to visit this part of Nepal while I was there. If other women were thinking of coming to Tansen, I thought the civil war and the previous Maoist attack must have scared them off, but I never really knew. From my perspective Tansen appeared eminently safe for a woman, despite all the State Department hype. Padma was planning to visit her relatives in India after Tansen before heading to the UK to resume school in the fall.

Padma was the same age as my younger daughter, and had sparkling eyes along with a beautiful mocha complexion. She was very intelligent but careful never to speak too soon. At the dinner table we learned that her avowed goal was to become a pediatric oncologist. I found myself thinking about the altruism of youth, especially among young medical professionals that were contemplating life's path. She seemed sincere and ingenuous. Over the whole summer I don't think she ever said one sarcastic thing.

Padma had traveled through a dozen European countries, and she knew her friends would want her to compare Tansen to the places she had been, so when we discussed Tansen I had this idea that she was rehearsing the comparison in her mind. She compared it to Italy. We decided that we were actually in the Poor Man's version of Tuscany – the Tuscany of Nepal. Tansen was on a hill with picturesque buildings of the Newari period. It enjoyed a panoramic view of the large valley below and was above the area where malaria mosquitoes lived. From the hospital we could see loops of the road that zigzagged up hill to the town, and terraced rice paddies which were dry when I was there. The town included a maze of narrow streets where the eaves of the brick buildings nearly touched overhead and the children played in a street little more than an alley way wide. Even on sunny days these were shaded and cool and there would be knots of women sitting together on the stoop of each house.

Near the center of town, where Steep Street and Flat Street join, there is a short tunnel that leads from the *Bajar* to the east side of town. Hundreds of people use this every day. The person who showed it to me made an offhand remark saying the tunnel always reminded her of Jerusalem so for the rest of the summer we called it the Jerusalem Tunnel.

Nanglo's is the classiest restaurant in Tansen. It occupies a spot on the main square near the "Elephant Gate," where Flat Street and Steep Street join. Here the security guard is an imposing former *ghurka* wearing the dark green *gurkha* military uniform. The waiters wear matching vests and *topis* made of *Palpali Dhaka*. The menu is in English. Every *videshi* eats there at least once a month, and out of town guests are always brought there. In the open-air dining area, dozens of swallows flit overhead as the sun goes down, and Nepali traditional music plays in the background. An outdoor sink is prominent on one wall, a feature of even the best Nepali restaurants, since so much of the Nepali cuisine is eaten with the right hand. Indoors, up a flight of stairs, is a place where you can sit on pillows Nepali-style, or perhaps look out the window in the old-fashioned *Newari* pastime of gazing discreetly at passersby. On the third floor the tables are higher and you can sit in chairs. Nanglo's is the outpost of a popular Kathmandu restaurant of the same name.

Like a hill town in Tuscany, Tansen has cobblestone streets. Cows, water buffalo, and pigs wander the streets. The climate is sunny and warm. Instead of vineyards there are terraced rice paddies. The colorful local characters include Magar women in their distinctive attire and diminutive male porters in short pants hefting impossibly heavy loads on a tumpline. Near the *Bajar* is a neighborhood where groups of men always play *carom*, a sort of billiards using checkers on a table-sized game board dashed with talcum powder, hens and chicks running underfoot. Young boys watch and the women sit nearby, three generations together. A continual cricket or soccer match plays out on the *Tundhikel*, the parade ground at the base of the town. There are no lawn mowers, instead people with sickles collect the grass as fodder and bring it home to feed goats tethered outside houses. When there is a bare patch of ground, it is planted with maize, even if it is next to the *Bajar*.

A westerner can walk through the Tansen *Bajar* as if he or she is invisible. None of the Nepalis pay any attention, which is very different than Kathmandu or other parts of Nepal, where the hawkers zero in on tourists. The guidebook refers to Tansen as unspoiled. On the walk to town there are often women making bricks from sun-dried mud the way people must have done five hundred years ago, as well as people using hand looms to weave the local *dhaka* cloth, for which Tansen is famous. Groups of women and girls sit in the sun grooming each other's long black hair while some nurse babies. Local tailors work at foot-powered machines outside their shops, as do the barbers and cobblers. Tansen has a collection of human-powered cottage industries, and we all noticed the simplicity of the way business was conducted. This was a lot less expensive than Tuscany. *Ah, the high life!* No casual tourists ever got this far into rural Nepal.

In the cool of the evening, Tansen springs to life. During "load shedding" – the euphemism for a blackout – all the shops are lit by candles, lending a medieval air to the activities within. There are no street lights. The houses do not have curtains on the windows, and if a person is walking back to the hospital after an evening in town, it is easy and tempting to peer into the houses, to take in domestic scenes. An interior designer would say that the main mode of decoration was minimalist.

Some houses along the way to town have black fiberglass water tanks on the top floor, a sign that the owner receives a water delivery every week and has indoor plumbing. There are many houses that had no such water system. To get the water for these households is the women's job. The daily routine is to carry jugs to the local *dhara*, or water tap. This is a daily ritual in South Asia, and women carrying water jugs are a common sight. When a woman gets married, it is customary for the groom's family to buy her some new water jugs as a wedding present. When the children are old enough to walk, they too will bring water from the tap each day, even if it is only in a Pepsi bottle.

At each neighborhood tap, the women gather at six in the morning and fill their jugs. Depending on the size of the tap, the women will also bathe at this time, even though the water at the tap is not heated. The logic is simple: why haul the bath water all the way back to the house when you are going to use it right away anyway? So the bathers wear a *lungi*, a loose wraparound affair like a Hawaiian *muumuu*. It may be clingy, but it allows them to maintain modesty. A woman can soap up, scrub and rinse off while remaining clothed.

Men also bathe at the tap, and when they do they strip down to their underwear. It is not unusual to see a group of nearly naked men bathing with their backs turned to the women, while a group of women bathe and shampoo their hair wearing a wet clingy loose fitting garment.

Everyone averts their eyes. They pretend to be invisible to each other, and boundaries are maintained. When people were bathing, I always walked quickly past for fear of being accused of gawking.

After a few days of general hospital orientation at Mission Hospital, Padma decided to spend her time in the Maternity Ward. She briefly came down to the Medical Ward to see what was happening when we had our snakebite victim on the ventilator, but that was the only time she saw what I did at the hospital until her last day or two.

Still, I saw Padma nearly every evening at the dinner table in the Guest House, taking part in the daily bull sessions with the guys. Our first task was to check the sign-up sheet and see how many would be eating that evening. Dinner began promptly at six and not sooner, out of courtesy to those who might be coming directly from the clinic or Theater. We always saved a portion for any person who had signed up but who might be late. The main course was almost always a casserole in a large pan. To divide the pan up into the correct number of sections was next. If there are eight people you just make one lengthwise cut and three crosswise cuts to obtain eight equal portions. If there were seven people though, we would sometimes discuss the best way to divide the pan evenly into portions with the fewest cuts. It was a silly math problem involving prime numbers, but one to which we solemnly adhered. Padma would often do the honors of cutting once we had decided.

After dinner, the western medical students usually watched DVDs in the Guest House TV room, and Padma would be there with the guys. Early on, I would go to my apartment and get the cookies my *didi* had made, to share with the gang, along with powdered milk in cold water. After two weeks they learned that if they planned in advance, the Guest House *didi* would make them a wonderful chocolate cake for about two hundred rupees, which is about two dollars and seventy-five cents in US money. The med students were generous in sharing so a number of evenings I also joined them for cake.

The DVD library included only a few action movies. *Lord of the Rings* – we all thought that maybe we were in Middle Earth. The scenery, the costumes, the mixing of cultures, the ancient buildings, the languages, religions and customs – it all existed right here in Tansen. *We were in Middle Earth right now.* In the Tolkien books, the Shire was at one edge of the known world. *Mission Hospital was located where the world ended and where Middle Earth began.* We debated whether Tolkien could have visited Nepal and used it to inspire his books. *Shakespeare in Love* was a favorite, and again, we could see aspects of medieval culture that persisted here to this day. I told Padma that if I ever wrote a book about my time in Tansen, when the movie came I would reserve the role of Padma for

Gwenyth Paltrow. We all loved Gwenyth. I was a fool for any red haired woman – Kate Hepburn, Bonnie Raitt, Cate Blanchett, my former wife – but Gwenyth was in a class by herself.

At least three or four times a week, the town, the Guest House and the hospital would go dark. The *Chowkidar's* job was to manually restart the hospital generator, which sometimes took a few minutes while he walked to the switch. The Guest House was linked to the hospital. And so, we would sit awhile trying to decide whether to light a candle. We soon learned to just stay put and wait it out. After awhile we would hardly even stop talking when it went dark, acting as though nothing had happened. One time we continued eating nonchalantly, though we all knew that we were proving to ourselves how "cool" we could be. The only sound was the tentative clink of forks against dinner ware. We were all maintaining a beautiful decorum. *The Chowkidar was not walking too quickly this evening. How long can we keep this up?* There were sounds of suppressed laughter, like kids hiding in a closet during hide-and-seek.

After five minutes, Al said, "Please pass the salt" in an utterly deadpan way.

In an innocent voice, Padma used her best Mary Poppins accent as she chimed in, "Do you suppose this is what it is like to be blind?"

Another time we sat quietly on the pillows watching a DVD when the power went out. After a minute or two somebody farted like a tuba. We broke out in uproarious laughter. We never discovered who the culprit was.

Whenever a new mother was admitted to the Surgical Ward, Padma would visit as part of the entourage of the maternity team, as they made rounds. We always said hello but there was no time for much conversation beyond this. She was enjoying obstetrics.

If You'll Be My Bodyguard, I Will Be Your Long Lost Pal

The other medical student whose time in Tansen most closely overlapped with mine was Al McVain, who arrived before Padma did. There was a constant stream of people coming and going between Tansen and the outside world, and Thursday was the usual day of the week for people to arrive. The Buck left Tansen every Wednesday and returned with the new people the next day late in the afternoon. Every one had to tell the story of their trip on the Buck. If the Buck was late, everyone seemed to know.

For several weeks there was a rumor that a medical student from the UK would come in mid-June. Normally a single person would be assigned to the dorm section of the Guest House, in the main building, but there were too many singles already and he was a bit longer-term than the usual; he would be in Tansen for six weeks. My apartment was family-sized, meaning that there was a second bedroom with two bunk beds that I was not using. I told Ganesh that the UK student could stay with me as long as he did not mind being in the room with the bunk beds. We wondered how tall he was and whether he would object. It turned out not to be necessary. When he finally arrived, Al shared a different place with another med student from the US and I stayed alone.

The Guest House is not a single building; it is more like a collection of small brick buildings connected by cobble stone pathways, like an English country village. Some of the buildings are large enough for a family. There is a main hall with a wing that has a series of small rooms like a monastery, for overnight visitors. The main hall has a high ceiling and is imbued with the slightly rundown, lived-in feel that you expect to find in the fellowship hall of a long-established United Methodist congregation in Maine.

The floor of the main hall is polished concrete with throw rugs. In the front part of the room, overlooking a big picture window, are some wicker rocking chairs and low sofas. On a clear day there is a panoramic view of the valley below. The walls are lined with bookshelves. One side is devoted to fiction - mostly paperbacks. The other side displays a collection of books about Nepal, as well as self-help books that seem to share a theme of good parenting and family adjustment. Travel guides. A basket of old magazines such as you might find in any doctor's office. On the coffee table is the latest edition of the *Kathmandu Post*. The main redeeming feature of the *Post* is that it is in English. The front page carried news of local disasters - bus accidents, floods, crop failures. Then political news. Otherwise, the entertainment section of the Post carries news of Paris Hilton and other Hollywood celebrities, a bit out of place in Tansen.

Away from the picture window in the back part of the main room are three dining tables that seat ten each. On one wall of this side are many books with Christian themes. Over the years, missionaries who brought these books left them behind when they moved on *like crutches piled outside the shrine at Lourdes.* On a small table below the bulletin board is the date book in which people reserve their seat at the dinner table. Pencil in a reservation before four PM. Flip through it and see who else will be around the table that night. On the other wall is the window into the kitchen, along with the supplies to make tea. The Guest House is chemical free apart from caffeine. On the far wall is a wooden plaque that reads:

CHRIST
is the unseen head of this household,
The guest at every meal,
A listener to every conversation

Each night there were between three and ten people around the table promptly at six. The first night Al arrived we heard a bit of his story. He planned to finish his degree, then take a year off to do biological research on cancer cell rejection. Following that, he would choose a residency and specialize. He had not chosen an area of specialty yet. Naturally we teased him about choosing gynecology.

"I don't think my girlfriend would approve," he replied, "and besides, I am painfully shy around women." The first day he joined rounds, he wore a white lab coat with the *Oxford Handbook* in one pocket – *"The Cheese and Onion"* as it is called. Soon he was just wearing a plain shirt like the Nepali interns and residents.

Al had bright blue eyes and blond hair, with a very pale complexion that did not get a tan. He was quick with a snappy comeback or a joke and knew a million stories, which he delivered in a British accent using slang that almost seemed like it was a put-on. He was also a good listener and seemed to always know just the right thing to say to somebody else to draw a good story out of them.

For the early part of the summer, Al chose to be on the surgical team, and I would see him every morning at surgery rounds. Then he would check the operative schedule, change into green hospital scrub clothes, and observe in Theater. In the afternoon he would change back into street clothes and go to the outpatient clinic. Al would also be involved in the preoperative workup of patients. It was a full schedule. He was the only medical student on the surgery team, however, and this meant he was the least senior person there. During ward rounds he was expected to tag along quietly and mainly listen.

Al's first impression of medical care in Nepal was a bit of a surprise to me. He said, "I underestimated the degree to which every patient here gets a thorough workup. I suppose I was thinking we just handed out the medicines when people asked for them. In fact, each patient gets a history and physical just as thorough as they would receive in the UK. The difference is, we have fewer X-rays and fewer lab tests available. Here in Tansen we probably depend on the history and physical exam more than they do in the UK."

Surgery Rounds

For the next three weeks, the leader of the surgery team would be Mark Powell, from the UK. Mark Powell was finishing up a year as a medical missionary and would be returning to England the first of July. Mark was thirty-five-years old and had completed most of his surgical residency at London with only a year to go when he decided to go to Nepal. After Tansen, he would return to the UK for his final year of training. His wife was a doctor also but mainly spent her time in Tansen as a stay-at-home mother to their three young children. When I heard Mark speak, I always thought of Tony Blair, the former British Prime Minister. Mark was tall and blond and always had a quizzical look about him. He was joined by Roger Lewis, a short-term volunteer surgeon from Scotland.

Surgery rounds are a daily ritual at Mission Hospital, practiced there in a form that anybody in Boston or London would recognize. In the morning, the team is joined by the charge nurse. The senior surgeon leads the rounds like the presiding judge in a county courthouse, or maybe the prosecuting attorney. The caravan is led by a wheeled wooden cart, in which the medical records of patients as well as x rays are ceremoniously stacked. The team stands at the foot of the bed as an intern introduces the case. The history is recited in a formal way. The surgery is reviewed. The patient is examined. The leader of the team gives verbal orders to the charge nurse who records them in a small notebook; and also dictates a progress note to a junior member of the team who writes in the chart. Then on to the next. Usually surgery rounded on about forty or so patients, not including those on Pediatrics, and orthopedic surgery rounded on fifty or sixty more.

I brought a very nice "torch" to Nepal, with a half-dozen fresh replacement batteries. I was in the habit of bringing it along on surgery rounds. With only a couple of bare bulbs in each room, the light on the Surgical floor depended on the patient's proximity to the window. As they made their way from one patient to the next, the surgeons would remove the dressings and inspect each patient's wounds. I would step forward and shine my nice bright torch. At first the surgeons would politely thank me. They soon got used to having this luxury and would direct me where to shine it for the best view. After Al arrived, he would hold the torch. We soon had a system so that when the Surgical Team arrived, Al would make hand signals for me to give him the torch. He came back to return it every day when rounds were finished.

Al was trying to learn as much about surgery as he could. At the dinner table we would discuss cases. Over the course of years watching ward rounds, I learned to appreciate rounds like it was a sports event or impromptu theater. It was a time to learn about the personalities of the team – who was clever; who could be trusted; who had a sense of humor, and so on.

Abdominal surgery was common at Tansen – gallbladders, appendixes, and intestinal surgery. Mark Powell also did gynecological surgery such as caesarean deliveries and hysterectomies. These would be typical of any general surgeon's practice in the West. Mark also did skin grafting for the burn victims, urological surgery, and thoracic cases. He occasionally did neurosurgery as well, when needed for trauma. I was impressed when I saw the surgical repair he had accomplished on a patient with Fournier's Gangrene, a tropical condition not often seen in the West. Fournier's Gangrene occurs on the scrotum, and can lead to loss of the testicles. I never heard of it before, and this was the first time I ever saw a patient after surgery to reconstruct the scrotum. Mark was versatile.

One morning the team was looking at an emaciated man about thirty-years old who had diarrhea. They were discussing typhoid or other causes of gastroenteritis. None of the suggested diagnoses seemed to quite fit, but the patient improved overnight after getting several liters of intravenous fluid and was less dehydrated than he had been. From the back row I quietly said, "Anybody check a T-3 cell count on him?"

Mark said, "Point well taken," but then ordered something else. I thought Mark completely ignored me, but on the way to the next patient he quietly said, "Joe, the euphemism we use for AIDS around here is 'B-24.' That was the first thing that crossed my mind yesterday when he was admitted, but this man does not have AIDS that we can tell."

Early on, I made sure to sit across from Mark at the dinner that followed one of the English-language services. I asked him about the range of surgery he performed.

He replied, "There are really only two surgical specialties at Mission Hospital – one is orthopedics. The other is – everything else!"

I asked Mark whether he thought a prospective surgeon would be interested in the cultural aspects of being in Nepal.

He replied, "Well, it's the country that never invented the wheel."
Whatever that meant.

As we ate our meat and potatoes, it seemed natural to talk about what the patients ate. Nutrition is important in postoperative healing. Mark said that each plate of *dal-bhaat* was about eight hundred calories, and the average Nepali got two plates a day, for a total of sixteen hundred calories. The diet is mostly carbohydrates and does not include much protein. Some of these patients would not have much nutritional reserve to promote wound healing after a major operation.

In the UK or US obvious trauma cases go to a surgeon. But every one else is examined by an internist, a non–surgeon, before a surgeon is called. The surgeon comes in to review the case only after the screening is largely completed. In Tansen, a patient gets a relatively brief screening in the ER or outpatient clinic, and then is sent to Medical or Surgical after this elementary *triage*. There is more responsibility on the surgeon to do the beginning workup, and to decide whether to treat an illness with a nonsurgical approach. In Nepal, the lack of resources makes it very important for the surgeon to consider whether the patient will survive the surgery. Mark was brilliant at this. When he led rounds he always considered the ethical implications that guided whether to perform surgery in rural Nepal.

Since Mission Hospital is a training center for Nepali doctors to become generalists, Mark supervised their learning in surgical skills. When he first took over, Mark identified the need to improve manual dexterity and suturing speed. He then arranged for each intern to spend time with pieces of buffalo, or pigskin, on a wooden frame, practicing their suturing skills. This was an innovation, and Mark was remembered as a taskmaster.

One morning before rounds, Mark and Roger Lewis were alarmed to look at the Theater schedule posted on Surgical. One of the young surgical residents was in charge of scheduling, and nine herniorraphies were on the list for the day. Nine men skipped breakfast and were waiting. Mark and Roger looked at the schedule and were furious. They did not want to do hernia surgery all day. They called the resident over and asked him how long he thought each of those was going to take? Did he know this was an hour apiece? That they would be doing hernias until 8 PM? The two surgeons interrogated the resident on the spot as to the signs of hernia and the indications for operation. That morning, they made the resident examine every single pre-op hernia patient as they went along. They were merciless. The female surgical resident was part of the group. Each time her rival was put on the spot, she seemed to be doing a little dance step right where she stood. She could not control herself. About half the patients were told to go home and come back another day.

I did not immediately meet Mark's wife Sandy. She had volunteered to join a two-week medical expedition to Mugu, a truly remote area of Nepal as part of a UMN outreach effort. At least once a month, Mission Hospital would gather a team of twenty or so people and send them out on four-wheel-drive vehicles to some far corner of the region. They would spend the weekend and examine four or five hundred patients. So the idea of sending people to conduct a remote clinic was not new, but the trip to Mugu was in a class by itself for distance and remoteness. Every two years, UMN would organize a self-contained surgical team, and charter a plane to fly them to Mugu, a remote town located at eleven thousand feet elevation in the Himalayas. While Sandy was gone, Mark watched the kids at night and a *didi* took care of them during the day – a Nepali Nanny.

One evening at the Guest House dinner table we were joined by Ellie, one of the Aussie doctors. He lived with his family about a mile away, but this evening Ellie was on call for the maternity department. When I first met him I pointed out that I did not know many men named Ellie, and he replied, "It's an old family name. 'Ellie' is short for 'Ellen' which is short for 'Lleweyllen'."

One of the American med students said that someday, he would like to volunteer with Doctors Without Borders, an NGO famous for sending medical teams to war zones through out the world. Ellie took another sip of tea and savored it in his mouth for a bit.

Here is what he said. "I know a lot of people who have done mission work all over the world, and I myself was in Somalia back in 1992 when it was a rough place. My advice to you would be to look very carefully at Doctors Without Borders. A friend of mine worked with them in Africa, and he said that when the volunteers were not doing clinical work, they were expected to find their own lodging and live directly with people from the community who would have them. They had to make their own arrangements to get food. This seriously impacted their ability to focus on their mission, and was not the best use of their specialized skills." The information was sobering. I thought of my *didi* and all the work she did. We all knew how much we depended on the staff of the Guest House."

"Choose your NGO carefully," he continued. "While it might appear that my stay was arranged by UMN, which is the International NGO that runs Mission Hospital, it was actually arranged by a sending organization in Australia. Both UMN and my sending agency treat me like I am family. I know all the people in the office and get excellent support. You are in the host country to deliver the best medical care you can. Don't underestimate the need for support."

Dessert that evening was chocolate cake, using Cadbury's chocolate. The *didis* at the Guest House did not usually make it with frosting. After dinner, I went back to my apartment to study for my language lesson while the medical students sat in front of the DVD player to watch *Speed*, starring Sandra Bullock.

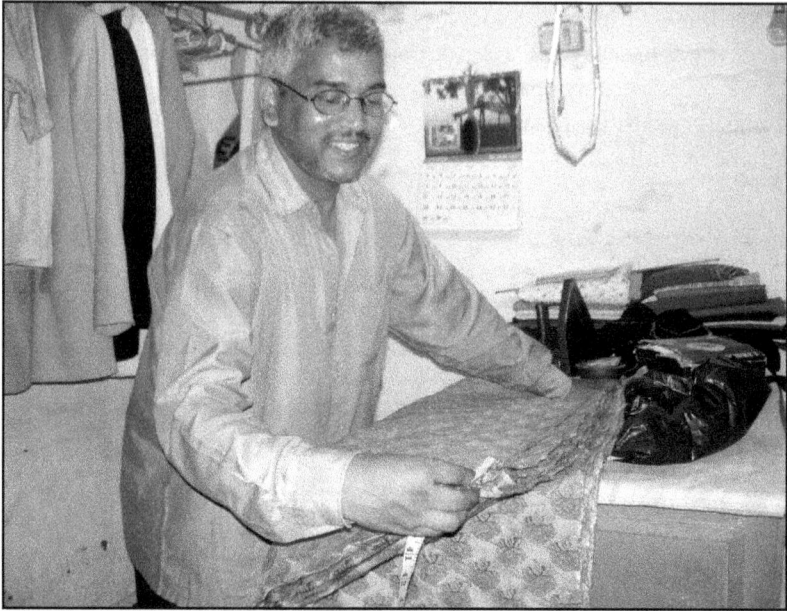

Kusiram at work, measuring
Dhaka cloth for a garment.

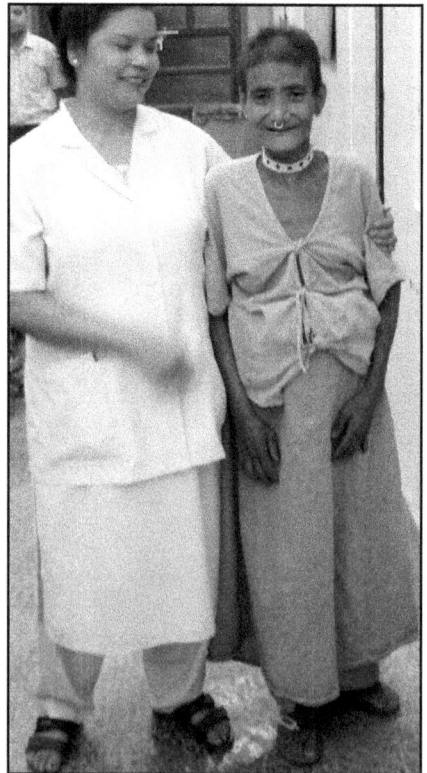

Answering the question, "What does a
modest Hindu lady wear in the hospital
when the American-style gowns would
be considered indecent?" Why, a two-
piece gown with a wraparound skirt, of
course.

Dressing and Looking the Part of a Magar Hill Woman

A *sari* is a piece of cloth six meters long. Girls start wearing a *sari* at around the age of fifteen, and it takes lots of practice to learn how to make the pleats in front correctly, otherwise the woman will not have the fluidity and grace that makes a *sari* so wonderful to wear. The colors of a *sari* are bright, usually some shade of red, pink or electric purple. An inexpensive cotton *sari* might be purchased for as little as a hundred rupees; a person wishing to go all out might pay thousands for a silk one with gold embroidery. Part of the *sari* goes over the shoulder and there are many ways to adjust it for comfort – on a cold day it is worn like a shawl, on a warm day it can be tossed over one shoulder. A Bollywood actress might wrap it low around the waist, showing her navel and hips, but here in Tansen it was more likely to be modest, covering everything but the hands and face. A *sari* is always worn with a short sleeve blouse that may show the midriff.

A *kurtha surwal* is also known as a *punjabi*, a sort of a pantsuit. The top extends to the mid-thigh or knee, and may or may not have long sleeves. It also comes with a narrow shawl which can be worn a number of ways to adjust to the sun or wind. Usually women wore bright color combinations. Often I saw women attired in a colorful *kurtha surwal* doing manual labor such as making bricks or shoveling. Because this kind of clothing was so modest, western missionary women dressed this way to fit in with the locals. The only exception was Doctor Norma, who always wore khaki pants and a casual button-down shirt.

There is no place to buy a *kurtha surwal* off the rack. In the *Bajar* in Tansen there are many tailors. On nice days, they work in the doorway of their shop, one foot pumping the treadle, enjoying the sunlight. Some of the sewing machines are fifty-years old, and there is one shop where the owner specializes in repairing these machines, sitting barefoot amidst a cool concrete floor strewn with odd parts like an auto junkyard. It is customary for the customer to buy the cloth and bring it to the tailor. He will make something from the cloth of your choice in two or three days. Kusiram is located about halfway down Steep Street in the *Bajar*. Because he speaks English he is the tailor favored by most women in the missionary community.

Very few women wear western style clothes. Saturday is the day off for the nursing students, the most westernized group of women in Tansen. In the morning they put on makeup and eyeliner, wiggle into their best designer blue jeans, maybe their only pair, and go to the *Bajar* in groups of two or three. I do not think I ever saw local women in western costume apart from this. One Saturday I ran into three of my students dressed in jeans, wearing makeup, and stopped to speak to them in the street. Within sixty seconds, a half-dozen men gathered around, wondering what was going on. *Maybe they were protecting the honor of these girls.* They seemed to be watching the women intently as we spoke. The women did not acknowledge that anything was unusual.

By far, the most interesting clothes are those worn by the hill people, the Magars. Their clothes are distinctive, and they always seem to carry the woven pack-basket of Nepal, known as a *dhoka*. On any given day, the stream of traffic through the *Bajar* includes groups of two or three Magar women trudging along, speaking among themselves, each one carrying a packbasket full of goods to bring back to their village, both hands near their ears to steady the *tumpline* that winds around their forehead to take the weight of the basket. From the beginning I thought to myself *they look like the hippie back-to-the-land women of Maine.* If the Magars had been transported to Maine, I could picture them burning cordwood to get through a Maine winter, driving an old beat-up car, growing their own food, and resisting commercialization. In Maine, the best single gathering place for such people is the Common Ground Fair, which is a tribal gathering for organic farmers and aging hippies every Fall before it gets cold. *The Bajar reminds me of the Common Ground Fair.* Both events convey the same makeshift jumbled crowd-of-people-but-not-sure-what's-going-on feel.

These Magar women are even more rugged than Mainers – in some cases their village might be several days' walk before they get to a paved road, and the women did not come to the *Bajar* often. *I wonder if they are wearing "gum rubbers,"* the term used by many people from Maine to refer to the rubber-soled leather boots from LL Bean. It would not have surprised me to see these. The older Magar women also wear a special gold jewelry piece in the septum of their nose, dangling over their lips, along with a side piece through the left *nares*. These are made of gold and handed down from mother to daughter.

I decided to send a complete set of Magar women's clothes to my daughter, the hippie organic farmer. Then I decided it would be great also to bring a set of clothes when I gave talks on Nepal. It would be a fine tool to engage the audience, augment my slides and give a feel of the experience to an American audience. The plan got more grandiose and ultimately I decided to buy four sets of clothes – one for each of my daughters, one for my former wife so she would not feel left out when the daughters wore theirs, and one to have at the University when I gave a talk on the experience. This project was not going to be accomplished with just one trip to the *Bajar*. I would need to overcome my shyness in dealing with the merchants at the *Bajar*. Here is what the well-dressed Magar woman wears. Start with a petticoat. This is a section of unhemmed cloth two meters long, usually of a bright color which does not have to match the skirt. Wrap it around the waist, and if it is too long, fold over the top part. Tuck the petticoat in on itself to hold it in place. Over the petticoat goes a skirt. I saw skirts in many colorful designs. The skirt is usually wide enough to go twice around the waist. As with the petticoat, if the there is too much material, fold the upper part, doubling it up.

Next is the *cholo*, the blouse. The distinctive feature of this is a double-breasted effect over the bosom, which is ideal for a breastfeeding woman. The preferred cloth for is *Palpali Dhaka*, a distinctive weave that is made locally by people using hand looms. There are a variety of patterns of *dhaka* cloth, in abstract geometrical shapes. *Dhaka* cloth is one of Tansen's main exports, and there were factories in town where the women sat at looms that looked as if they were made in 1820, operating the equipment with their feet and hands, silent except for the clacking and the songs of birds outside. A *cholo* is fastened with ties instead of buttons. There are four grades of *dhaka* cloth, and if the cheap *dhaka* cloth is used, the *cholo* must be lined. A Magar hill woman does not wear a bra or undershirt. Trust me. Far and away the most unusual item is the *patuka*, or belt. A *patuka* is five meters long – fifteen feet – and winds around the waist six or seven times, concealing the contour of a woman's belly. It is twisted willy-nilly as it is wrapped around the outside of the skirt and the *cholo*. The end is tucked in on itself. The Magar hill women use the last few folds of it to hold their money purse or other objects. The favorite color for a *patuka* is bright banana yellow. Every bona fide hill woman also carries a small sickle. If there is some tall grass along the way, she might stop, harvest some, and throw it in to the basket to bring back to the goat tethered by her house. The sickle is tucked into the *patuka* in the back.

No ensemble would be complete without a *potey* – a necklace – and a hair tassel. Women wear three or four necklaces, and again, these do not match in any conventional sense. The most prized *poteys* are made of bright green glass with beads the color of new rice shoots, worn by married women. The more strands on the necklace, the more expensive it will be. A hair tassel is made of red strings, and braided into the hair, giving the illusion of waist length hair. Magar hill women do not wear lipstick or makeup. They have a healthy glow about them. They smell like wood smoke.

Finally the shawl is a cherished item for all women. A shawl is worn regardless of the weather. In Tansen, the favorite style is very plain, a solid color with just a few hand-embroidered flowers or birds. A shawl lasts forever. A young woman is likely to own a less expensive cotton shawl, while an older woman would own one made of *pashmina*, the fine wool like cashmere. Everyone told me I needed to go to Pokhara to find a shop that sold *pashmina*.

After Clinical one day, I went to Kusiram, the tailor on Steep Street. It was a sunny day, and he was sitting behind his treadle-powered machine at the front of the shop, enjoying the bright sunlight while he worked. I asked him about *cholos*. He was just about my age but his hair was salt-and-pepper gray, a sharp contrast to his dark complexion. He told me okay, but there was one little problem. What sizes did I want? I could tell him the American dress sizes for each of the people on my list, but in Nepal they do not use the American numbering system. He showed me pattern books from the UK, Germany and Sweden, but he did not own any from the US.

Kusiram was incredulous that somebody would order a garment without knowing the size of the person who would wear it. "What are we to do?" He got out from behind his sewing machine and we stood together in the doorway to his shop on Steep Street, while he pointed his arm at passing women.

"Is that one about the size of your daughter? How about that one? Bigger? Maybe like Doctor Norma? Big like you? Or just bigger than that lady?" We decided that I would get just one at first. Maybe I could get somebody to try it on and see whether to make more.

Rescuing Patients

The third-year nursing students were eager to work in the Critical Ward on Surgical. I spent part of the time with the third year group and for them I had a very different approach than I did with the first year students. The first year students were learning the tasks of patient care, and going by the checklist to guide them about what to do next. It was a mechanistic way to get organized, but beginners have to start somewhere.

A third year student would soon graduate in about four months and take on more responsibility. An independent practitioner needs a level of thinking beyond simply making sure that the tasks are done. The student needs to learn how to manage a patient who is unstable.

Senior students need to learn how to "rescue" a patient from complications of surgery. To the layman, the surgeon gets all the credit for healing a person who has had an operation. But if the person did not get nursing care after the surgery, he or she would die. There are known complications of surgery and it is the nurse's job to identify them and take action to correct the problem.

Compared to the American patients I worked with, the Nepali patients did not get much pain medicine and they complained a lot less. I don't really know why they were so tough. We rarely worried about overdosing them on the pain medicines they were given.

One day we took care of a man who was post-operative from gallbladder surgery the day before and was in acute pain. They gave him two milligrams of morphine through the IV. His pain was much better. Five minutes later, though, he was unresponsive, and his breathing was labored. The nursing staff thought his breathing was about to stop altogether, so they put him on oxygen, prepared to intubate him and called the doctor. Before the doctor came, I took a closer look at him and noticed that his pupils were pin point. His breathing was slow and irregular. It was easy to conclude that he had been overdosed on morphine. When the doctor arrived I asked for a narcan order, the antidote to morphine overdose. The doctor agreed. We gave the drug and the change was dramatic. The man was fully awake within a minute or so and was able to breathe again.

His instantaneous recovery seemed miraculous to the Nepali nurses, who were not used to seeing patients with morphine overdose. They did not use narcan very often, if at all. I, however, was surprised that such a small dose of morphine would have caused this problem, especially considering the surgery the man had just had. In any case, the doctor thanked me and I heard later that he had told the other surgeons that I had made a good call.

A post-op patient will resist getting out of bed and standing up because it hurts, but lying still will cause pneumonia to develop. We made sure to assist the patients in turning from side to side instead of lying on their back all the time. I taught the students to use their hands to make a rhythmic cupping on the patient's chest to loosen the phlegm – a procedure known as chest physiotherapy; and showed them how to teach the patient to hold their belly when they coughed so it would not hurt so much. We needed to make this a priority, and I talked about it every morning, and then checked to make sure the students were following through. This was old-fashioned nursing care, but it made a big difference. Patients were less likely to run a fever.

In the US, the patients would be given a one-person-use plastic device called an Incentive Spirometer to promote lung expansion. We did not have any at Mission Hospital. I asked about just getting a few from the US, and then getting a system to clean and re-use them. They told me this idea had been considered but there was so much TB around that sterility could not be guaranteed if this kind of plastic device was reused from one patient to the next. So the answer was no, for a very good reason. This device, simple as it was, would be an unsustainable expense at Mission Hospital.

I did not know anything about Kala-Azar when we first cared for our man who had it. The third-year student assigned to him was named Sikha, and I told her that she needed to learn about the disease. Strangely the Nepali nursing textbook did not cover it, though Kala-Azar is common in Nepal, one of the top four countries in the world for visceral leishmaniasis. In the Medical Library I found a Tropical Diseases book that devoted a chapter to Kala-Azar. I photocopied the pages on the disease and gave them to Sikha, telling her I would quiz her the next day. I saw her first thing the next morning and pulled her aside. She started to tell me what she had learned – and it soon became clear that she could recite the whole chapter from memory backwards and forwards. I was pleased and surprised.

As soon as you walked into the men's ward you would notice Sargit, because his bed was right by the door. He was seventeen-years old and had fallen out of a tree while cutting the branches for firewood. His x-ray showed a clear fracture of the spine in his neck. He was barely old enough to shave and was now a partial quadriplegic. He could not move his legs, and his arms were weak. In order to stabilize his spine, this young man needed to be immobile for six weeks, using a device called "halo traction." The halo drew your attention. It gets its name from the way it circles the skull like a steel halo. Through it are four screws that fasten it to the skull sort of like a thorny crown. To provide traction, a hanging weight is attached via a rope and pulley. If we let Sargit lay flat all the time, he would develop bedsores, so I taught the first year students to turn him from side to side using a technique called "logrolling." A team of staff would carefully maintain body alignment so as not to jerk his neck while repositioning him.

He was not our only woodcutting injury. More commonly we admitted people with supracondylar fractures of the elbow. It was illegal to cut down trees for firewood. Nepal is being deforested and this leads to erosion, landslides and floods. I was looking around a hardware store one day and realized that you could not buy a chainsaw anywhere in the whole country. Then I looked for handsaws and I never found any place that sold those either. When I realized this I thought back to the State of Maine, and a friend who owned about six chainsaws as well as a skidder. *Bob Donovan would starve in this country*, I thought to myself. But it is not illegal to take some branches from a tree. So people climb up and get them. As the trees lose their branches, people have to climb higher and higher. They use a *khukri* to cut the branches. Somebody told me this but I did not believe them until one day I was walking in the woods above the hospital. In the distance was the sound of methodical chopping, like a huge woodpecker. I followed the sound to see a man collecting tree branches as they dropped, and craned my neck. The man doing the work was about forty feet up, whacking away with a *khukri*. I could barely make him out. *No wonder people break something when they fall from these heights. Is it better to break your elbow, or to snap your neck?*

It was not unusual to see groups of people returning to town from a trip to the nearby broadleaf forest, carrying bundles of wood on their back. One time I saw a young boy carrying a good sized log. He could not have been more than eleven-years old, but he hefted a hunk of wood that might have weighed seventy-five pounds. For some reason I found myself humming a hymn, *The Old Rugged Cross*, as I watched him trudge past. When they got home they would pile their firewood on the corrugated tin roof of their house where it would be out of the way while it dried.

Sarjit, the young man in halo traction, was a Muslim. There was a small community of Muslims in town, with an active Mosque, and more in the countryside west of Tansen. He was the sole support of his mother. She was about thirty-five and always wore a faded canary-yellow sari with abstract blue designs on it over a black blouse. The only skin she showed was that of her face and hands. She would climb on the bed with him and relentlessly work on range-of-motion exercises so that his muscles would be preserved if he should ever regain the ability to control them. When I walked by the bed, she would bring me over and show him to me. She thought I was one of the doctors since I was Caucasian. I asked a student to explain to her who I was and what I did there.

After three weeks of traction, the day came when the doctors on morning rounds felt Sargit was as healed as he could be, and there was no further therapy the hospital could offer. They told his mother that he would never recover. She threw herself at their feet in a dramatic scene. She wept. After that she worked even harder on the range-of-motion exercises, hoping against hope that he would recover through some miracle. In the long run, her son would need to go somewhere for long term care. She seemed to be in a state of chronic sorrow. I did not know what to say to her each day, other than a polite *Namaste*.

That evening Al called me a "bloke" at dinner. Sounded more like "Blowk" actually, but I was getting used to his accent.

"Hold it right there. I need clarification. When you say I am a bloke, what does that mean, exactly?"

"Don't worry, Joe, there is nothing wrong with being a bloke."

"Maybe, but I need a working definition here."

"Let's see, a bloke is a regular guy, one you might find in a pub minding his own business, but usually pretty solid, the kind of guy you can trust. Since that man with Buerger's Disease, I have thought of you as a bloke. "

"Thank you. So you are telling me there is no negative connotation to the word?"

"That would be correct. Now, as a bit of advice, never ever, under any circumstances, allow a person to call you a 'lad.' Being 'one of the lads' is not a desirable state."

"What about 'chap'?"

"Nobody says 'chap' anymore, my friend."

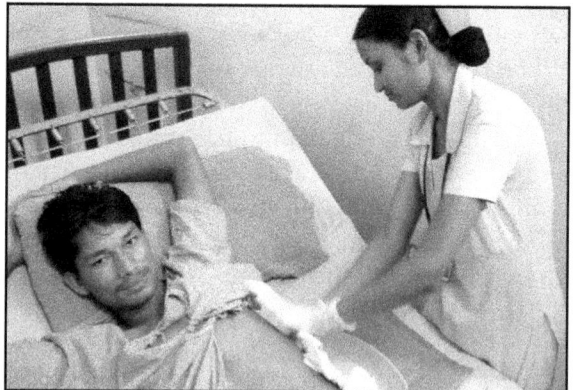

TNS student performing dressing change on patient in Critical Ward. American nurses do not generally wear the traditional nurses cap. clean gloves such as she is wearing are sent to be washed and reused until they break.

Maternity and Nativity

Around this time, Padma was spending every waking moment studying obstetrics. She divided her time between outpatient, inpatient and postpartum. She had learned how to check a cervix, I could sometime see her waving two fingers in the air like imaginary scissors, and I would chuckle at the recognition that she was processing her new found skill. She was now able to track the progress of labor, and evaluate the mother. At the dinner table, we were incredulous when she reported that she had seen an eight-year old boy take a mouthful of breast milk from his mom while they waited to see the mom's new baby in the postpartum clinic. And she also told us more about childbirth in rural Nepal.

The Maternity Ward at Mission Hospital was not a place where I had much business. I knew that men did not attend childbirth in Nepal. This is true even for the father of the baby. Women don't attend cremations; men don't attend childbirth. A simple system. In the geographic area served by Mission Hospital, there were ten thousand deliveries a year, but only fifteen hundred took place in the hospital. The vast majority of babies were born at the mother's home. In a high percent of cases, this really meant that the home delivery took place in a cowshed behind the family farmhouse.

Whoa. It sounded strange to me at first. Many of the houses in Palpa district were constructed of sun-dried bricks made of mud that was usually dug up right on site. In such a house there would be a dirt floor, reinforced by cow manure to give the walking surface a springy smooth appearance. It is porous. If you have ever been around during a delivery, you know that when a baby is born, he or she is accompanied by at least a few liters of the mother's amniotic fluid and blood. If a woman delivered the baby in the house, all these body fluids would drip onto the floor, and soak in. The only way to clean the floor is to get a shovel and dig up the floor. By contrast, if the woman delivers the baby in the shed, the body fluids are be absorbed by the straw, which is a lot easier to replace. So I suppose that was the logic. The obvious problem with giving birth in the shed is lack of hygiene. Over a five year period the government and public health groups succeeded in decreasing the number of women giving birth in the shed. The government was also trying to decrease the incidence of neonatal tetanus.

When I heard about the cowshed issue, it made me rethink the nativity of Jesus Christ. In Nazareth, it may have very well been the case that *every* woman in Biblical times gave birth in the stable. *The Bible* does not give the statistics to determine whether this was unusual or not. In the West, when the nativity is told, we hear the phrase "no room at the inn" and we are conditioned to feel sorry for Mary, as though Mary was being singled out, but maybe Mary was being treated the same as every other woman of her day.

The next thing Padma told me was that most forms of contraception only became legal in 2003. Adolescent pregnancy was widespread. On a walk to the *Bajar* there were always a number of teenaged girls carrying babies. I learned to look for the vermilion painted at the part of her hair near the forehead, and to try to estimate the age of the woman more closely. If the vermilion was there, she was married and the baby was hers, regardless of how young she may have looked. I wondered how old Mary was when Jesus was born.

In Nepal every nurse receives midwife training during their undergraduate education, and every nurse in Labor and Delivery was qualified to conduct a delivery. The doctors only got involved if there were complications or if a cesarean delivery was needed. Padma was hoping to deliver some babies this summer, and if it was going to happen, she would need to build the trust of the midwives first. She would also need to be assertive and find the right time to jump in and be in charge when the time came. She would need to work with the doctors as well. Padma had a lot on her plate. We were all hoping she would get her wish. Al told us about nearly dropping a baby when he did obstetrics; and we teased Padma about whether she would drop her first baby on the floor. They are slippery.

Missionary Comings and Goings

Mark Powell was leaving July 1st and we had a short-term coverage gap in *videshi* surgeons. This had been the cause for considerable discussion all Spring, but there had been no luck in recruiting. The administrators cobbled together a schedule of short-term surgeons. Roger Lewis, the seventy-seven-year-old retired Scottish surgeon, who had been with us for just a month, was going to Bangladesh for a prior commitment there. The hospital had even considered whether to relax the requirement that a long term volunteer surgeon be a Christian. Fortunately, Dr. Cooper from Australia was in Tansen for two weeks. There was an Indian surgeon now practicing in the UK named Hom, and he too would make a side trip in Tansen for two weeks with his family. In the meantime we would also have a surgeon named Park for a month.

I first met Park on a late Thursday afternoon within five minutes of the arrival of the Buck, and I assumed correctly that he had just arrived. He was rolling his luggage behind him – a set of matching black leather bags. Usually westerners were careful not to display many leather items in this cow-worshipping Hindu country, but here was a man who seemed to love leather. He was near the canteen, walking through the lower gate area where they were doing hospital construction, which was where the Buck stopped to disgorge passengers and cargo. Picking one's way through piles of gravel and stone, past the workers carrying material in baskets on their backs with a *tumpline* on their head, would have been disorienting for anyone. He was obviously new.

I saw him and went over to introduce myself but before I could speak he said, "I need to present my credentials to the hospital administrator – can you tell me where her office may be?"

I told him how to get to her office then I tried to introduce myself and shake his hand, but he ignored this gesture. Usually after a ten-hour ride through the Nepal countryside, the people that got off the Buck were tired but mellow. He was abrupt and a bit dismissive. It seemed odd that he might have not sent his credentials long before arriving, and odder still that this could not wait until morning.

Park was about thirty-two and wore glasses. He wore expensive leather shoes with pointy toes. His belt was leather. He had a dark dress shirt that would have looked in place at a disco, and pleated pants with a crisp front crease. *How did that crease survive the long trip on the Buck? It is a mystery.* He parted his hair on the side and had a shock of it that went all the way across the top of his head. I noticed his mannerism of flipping it into place every now and then, and he seemed to be always trying to put it back over his forehead with his hand. I knew older guys that did this to cover a bald spot but Park was not bald. Like many Asians, Park did not look like he needed to shave very often and I wondered if he shaved every day. If he did, he used an electric. I wondered if he brought it. He was shorter than I am and thin.

I learned later that he was from South Korea. He would be the senior surgeon once Mark Powell and Roger left. He signed up to do a yearlong medical mission to Afghanistan through a Christian NGO. *Afghanistan! Home of the Taliban, and a country at war.* Tansen had its limitations, but with a fifty-year history of hospital culture, this was paradise compared to Afghanistan. Park was likely to be putting himself at personal risk. The very idea was heroic. *Awe inspiring.* We already knew what it was like being here, with lots of support. For us, Tansen was challenging enough. *Afghanistan! Wow!*

He came to dinner at the Guest House the first evening but ate with another Korean who was there and did not speak to the rest of us. Within a day or two, we learned that Park had just finished his residency in a world-class, thousand bed medical center in Seoul, a sophisticated city of ten million people. It was only recently that he signed on to a Christian NGO for the Afghanistan mission. The leaders of his NGO told him he needed to be able to hit the ground running in Afghanistan, so they arranged with UMN for Park to orient by coming to Tansen for a month. For Park, Tansen would be a sort of transition or halfway house before the real deal.

It seemed very odd for Park to decide all this at the last possible minute. I learned later that he had not studied Afghanistan and knew very little about the country; he certainly had not studied Nepal or he would have gotten rid of the leather goods. He knew nothing of language or customs. I spent six months preparing to come to Nepal, and I was astounded that somebody would make a decision to do such a mission at the last minute.

We were accustomed to a high standard of surgical competence. Mark had been there a year. In addition to the surgery, Mark helped Krishna, the Chief of Surgery, with the training program for the junior house staff. Mark was a taskmaster, insisting that the junior staff practice suture technique. They could all do the one-handed knot right out of the World Health Organization textbook on surgery. He led the team and assigned roles to each intern. Mark led the morning rounds and was intelligent and compassionate.

The chief of surgery was Doctor Krishna, the Nepali orthopedic surgeon. Krishna was taking two weeks vacation in Kathmandu during Mark's last days. When Mark left, Krishna knew he would be losing a trusted right-hand man. Our other short-term surgeons were also leaving. Roger was heading to Bangladesh in another week and would spend the rest of the summer there. And the short-term orthopedic surgeon from Japan had one more week to go.

There would be a week of transition at rounds with Park joining the team before Mark left. On day one, Park stepped up to the bedside of the very first patient and removed the soiled surgical dressing. Park palpated the patient's surgical incision with his bare hands. Park waved off the clean gloves we offered him. The charge nurse and I looked at each other with surprise, because we knew that this was long-established practice here. What was more amazing was that instead of letting Mark and Roger lead the rounds, Park was vocal about asking questions and challenging the way that the IV fluids were ordered. He started to recite to Mark and Roger about the differences between Central Venous Pressure monitoring and Swan-Ganz catheter readings to determine fluid volume.

After a few moments of politely listening, Mark interrupted him, gave some orders to the junior intern, and moved to the next patient. Before he could touch the second patient with his bare contaminated hands, the charge nurse and I took Park aside, led him by hand to the portable sink and made him wash his hands. We told him to use gloves and handed him a pair.

The next patient had pancreatic cancer and jaundice. Mark had done a palliative biliary stenting to relieve the blockage of the duct. Once again Park started to show what he knew by pulling out a spiral-bound notebook and drawing a diagram to show Mark the technique to resect cancer of the head of the pancreas. Mark firmly stated that the object was not cure but palliation. Mark then added that we did not have the ability to do the kind of pancreatic surgery Park suggested, it was too risky. That silenced Park for about a minute.

On the third patient Park was re-stating his ideas on pulmonary artery wedge pressure monitoring. It seemed as though he did not quite grasp the need to focus on the actual person lying in the bed in front of him. Mark ended up being a bit more forceful in saying that he, Mark, would run the rounds this morning, and Park needed to see the way it was done before trying to use this as a platform to teach things that were not relevant.

I could see that this was not going well, and I thought *Am I the only one who thinks this is bullshit?* I looked around and I could see the reactions on the faces of the others on rounds. *They see it too.* As the surgical team moved on, I took Al aside and asked if he thought anything was strange about the way the new guy was acting. Al said he thought Park did not know when to stop talking.

At about two that afternoon I walked to the hospital canteen for a snack, and I saw the surgical team already there, enjoying some *chiya* on the wooden benches outside. I immediately noticed that Park was sitting on a bench slightly off by himself while the rest of the surgical team was at another table. I sat across from him and ordered some *momo* with *achaar*. I asked how things were going. He started to tell me he was amazed at the things that Mission Hospital did not have. *This is not a good way to start on your first day.*

I looked at him and said, "Park, I have worked with post-open-heart surgery patients and in major tertiary medical centers in the US. I know how to run hemodynamic monitoring and all the equipment you are talking about. This is not the place to do the fancy stuff, so I never talk about it here – that is a waste of time. I think you need to start with what you yourself need to learn." The *achaar*, when it came, was delicious, very subtle in spices. Sometimes they added ginger.

Park watched me eat for a minute and said, "But it's just not the way I was taught."

I said, "We have all made an adjustment when we got here. We are in a remote location in a country with lots of challenges, and I think it is miraculous what they do here. You need to learn new things, study it more."

Later that day I went to my room to find the copy of *Common Medical Problems in the Tropics* which I studied when I first arrived. *Maybe Park could benefit from this. It will help him "get hip."* I put the book in my daypack and brought it to Surgical. I asked around and found Park in the Recovery Room. As I handed him the book I said, "Park, maybe if you have been working in a referral center you are not as sure about the kind of primary care we are trying to deliver. Read this. It will help you make some sense about the practical aspects of what we are trying to achieve."

He took it and said, "Thanks." Somebody else had also given him *Surgery at the District Hospital*, a text from the World Health Organization.

Despite this, the next day was more of the same, and it was more obvious that the other surgeons were annoyed with Park. They were beginning to ignore any comments he made, and carry on the discussion as if he had not said anything. I knew what I had told Park, but he ignored it. Once more I stopped at the hospital canteen before going to my language lesson. The team was there for afternoon *chiya*, and I noticed that this time, Park was sitting further away. I sat with him as the others talked in low tones with their heads together. One or the other would put their head up and glance over every now and then. If they caught my eye they would arch their eyebrows quizzically. Park told me he felt he'd been humiliated. I told him that the way they did things here was backed up by a solid rationale and he should learn the rationale before criticizing. I asked him if he read the book I lent him, and he said, "No."

On the third day of rounds, Park suggested that we do exploratory abdominal surgery on the man with ascites. This was roundly rejected, and Park defended his idea by saying "It may even be at the risk of the patient's life," which resulted in some raised eyebrows and prompted a discussion of the limits of surgery. Mark seemed frustrated. *What part of shut up and listen does Park not get?* I thought to myself. Later, I saw Mark in the hall.

I told Mark that I had given Park the book, and that I did not think he had read it. "Park is not ready for Afghanistan," he told me curtly that day. "That's all there is to it. Somehow he does not want to learn what we are doing here."

I could not resist a sarcastic reply. "You know what his problem is? He does not know the facts of life if you asked me. We're all telling him stuff and he is ignoring it. He's acting like a twelve-year-old."

Mark looked into space for a second and I think he decided not to respond to my off-color remark, "I know," he said.

Park went to Theater the next day and looked over the shoulders of Mark and Roger while they did some routine cases. Maybe he was going to ease into things after all, and the Theater might be the place where Park could show his stuff. After talking with Mark, I tried to stay out of the surgical team's business. I did not want to appear as if I was piling on, did not want to drag the team even further down. But here they were, playing out a little interpersonal drama every day, with Park suggesting things that the others shot down immediately. At rounds, the nursing staff derives part of the game plan for each patient through the verbal instructions that are given. Here was a case where the verbal dialog was a mishmash of contradictory instructions, which can become troublesome for the nurses during the day as they carry out the medical plan. When things get this ragged, mistakes can be made. Life was already difficult enough.

The Last Night of the Proms

Saturday was the big day for Mark and his family. We would have a going away party after the English-language church service. The whole *videshi* community would be there. The *didis* of the Guest House would make a special meal. Extra tables were added. We all wondered what they would serve this time.

The surgical team was functioning with just the minimum crew since no surgery was scheduled for Saturday. Park was in charge of rounds that morning. I stopped by the ward before going to the library and church. Looking at the bottom edge of the curtain, I could see all their feet around a bed on the Gynae Ward, so I joined them behind the curtain. They were gathered around an elderly lady lying on her back who had a recent palliative mastectomy. She wore a kerchief over her hair. Her hospital gown had been slipped off her shoulder, and her arm raised, exposing the suture line where the breast had been. There was a boggy collection of fluid under her incision, which often happens with mastectomies since the lymph nodes are disrupted. A needle aspiration was called for.

The Nepali surgeons were trying to tactfully suggest that somebody return to Surgical after rounds to do this, but Park insisted that he do it on the spot. It took him twenty minutes while the other three stood there. They were whispering among themselves and pretending to look busy reading the chart of the next patient. The charge nurse was frowning because Park was not wearing gloves while he tried to suck the excess fluid out with the syringe, and when I pointed this out he said, "It will just take a minute, no need for gloves."

I went to the cupboard and got a pair and laid them down right next to his hands. He ignored the gloves and kept poking. I decided not to stick around. Later Al told me they did not finish rounds until eleven, an hour longer than usual.

That afternoon the English-language service was every bit as nice as we hoped. The furniture at the Guest House conference room was re-arranged in rows like a church would be, and the conference table was pushed out of the way. Everyone wore their best clothes including the children. Ellie showed up in a bow tie. Two of the doctors played electric piano and guitar. Hymns were chosen from the little yellow Aussie hymnal. There was something about the harmony and words of this songbook that always made me think we were in the Australian Outback. *The back of Beyond... the slang term for the Outback.... It also applies right here.*

The high point of the service came when everyone took turns to offer prayers for Mark and Sandy's journey. We gathered round the couple and put our hands on their shoulders. One by one, all the other *videshis* still serving in Tansen addressed the departing couple directly as they offered prayers for a good transition and reentry. I listened from the back row, and realized that if you turned it around, each prayer revealed their own future wishes for themselves when it would be their turn to go back to the world. As each person spoke, I found myself hoping they each would receive the same goodwill when they left, a sense of longing for good things to happen to people who had given so much.

I surveyed the room and noticed that Park was not there among us. At the end of the service, the children scooted out and the adults stayed in the conference room with the projector to hear Sandy, Mark's wife, tell about her trip to Mugu. She showed pictures of the equipment they brought, how they set things up, and who they saw in the clinic. We could see the faces of the women she met, while we heard their stories told by an articulate person who had been in Nepal for a year.

Then we gathered round the tables for a fried chicken dinner with mashed potatoes, along with green beans. The gravy was rich dark brown. The smell of coffee filled the room. A squadron of kids ran underfoot, playing hide-and-seek under the tables. I brought out my trumpet and played *For He's a Jolly Good Fellow, God Save the Queen,* and *Rule Britannia.* Mark was surprised that I knew the tune to *God Save the Queen.* I told him, every American knows that tune, but maybe not the same lyrics. Then *Auld Lyng Syne.* The afternoon was a fitting tribute to the family that was leaving. Every one had the opportunity to say a personal good-bye. There was spice cake with white frosting for dessert.

On Sunday in the late afternoon, the first day of the Nepali work week, Park did his first independent surgery. The patient was about sixty-years old, had a strong history of alcoholism and now had stomach pain due to an inflamed pancreas. In this patient the duct by which digestive juice flowed from the pancreas to the small intestine was blocked, causing a backup. It causes pain, and after a while scar tissue forms around it, which is known as a "pseudocyst." If the scar tissue is thick enough, the pseudocyst can be lanced, the fluid is drained, and then another adjacent opening can be created in the stomach. Then the two openings in the stomach and pancreas are joined together to form a new drainage route. This surgery is a major undertaking. Park took the patient to Theater with no assistant and with no consultation.

I was surprised on rounds Monday morning to see Mark appear on Surgical wearing the same off-white lab coat and checkered shirt I had seen so often. I said, "I thought you were outta here."

Mark looked at me, stood straighter and thrust his lower jaw forward. The effect was to look down his nose, something I had never seen him do. He paused and said, "I thought so too. I have been packing... I was called to put some things to right."

When Park appeared, Mark set his jaw and blushed. He curtly told the team to follow him to the first bed, where Park's patient awaited. At the foot of the first patient's bed, Mark stood toe to toe with Park and delivered a short and vehement lecture in which he bluntly and openly criticized Park for his lack of surgical judgment. Mark held the clipboard in one hand, stabbing it with the index finger of his right hand for emphasis as he spoke. Mark was red-faced and furious. Park cringed.

When Park attempted to fix the pseudocyst, he misjudged the degree of the scar tissue. When he got to the organ and incised it, Park discovered that the scar tissue was not thick enough to attach any sutures. Not even one stitch. Park panicked, did some unnecessary dissection, nicked the colon, and then actually left the OR without closing the patient. The anesthesia technician stood there, with the clock ticking, giving anesthesia to a patient with an open incision and no surgeon. The anesthesia technician decided to send a messenger to summon Mark away from packing his belongings. Mark walked in cold to finish the surgery that Park had started.

The pancreas produces a caustic fluid that digests food in the small intestine. If the fluid escapes into other parts of the abdomen, it can disrupt wound healing. And now we had a man who would inevitably develop a bellyful of pancreatic fluid in the wrong place. Mark was livid and the anesthesiologist refused to allow Park to set foot into Theater, let alone perform surgery. Later I found and read the patient's chart, and flipped through to find Mark's report from Theater. It was the most vivid and scathing progress note from a surgeon I had read in my whole career.

Mark told one of the Nepali surgeons to take charge of the team today, and then left. There was stunned silence among the surgical team. I followed Mark down the corridor for a bit and spoke to him as he stopped to wash his hands.

I said, "I don't know what happened with this patient. Are you telling me that Park intentionally botched this somehow?" As an afterthought it occurred to me that Mark was a Christian Missionary who probably did not think in these crude terms. "Sorry if the language offends you," I added.

Mark looked at me and said, "No, I am not offended. We need more of that kind of plain talk. There has not been enough. Go back and really look at that patient. The man in that bed was experiencing abdominal pain from pancreatitis which would not have killed him.

Park tried the surgery and the patient will die now, needlessly, because of Park's lack of judgment and skill. Somebody here will need to protect these patients from Park." Then he broke it off and stalked down the hall toward the administrator's office.

The surgical team carried on with ward rounds. The team was speaking to the patients, and to each other, in Nepali. *Brilliant. The best way to keep it focused.* I could follow the gist of what they were saying only because I could refer to my notes. If Al, the medical student from the UK, asked a question in English, somebody on the team would answer him in English. Park was now a nonexistent person and they were not subtle about refusing to speak to him. He stood on the outside row. He looked pale. This was the same day we had our snakebite victim come through the ER, so I rushed away in a hurry, and I did not witness the rest of the rounds.

I ate with the others at the Guest House that evening. We had lots to discuss since it had been an action-packed day for me. When the snakebite victim arrived, I had a full plate and the saga of Park became a sideshow – a distraction. I told Al at dinner that I had seen people shun a person, cutting them off from social reinforcement, but the degree to which Park had become a pariah was unparalleled in my experience.

"Let that be a lesson to you Al – in your own medical career – I hope that you never become the kind of non-person that Park has now become."

Al said, "Surely this fellow had these problems long before he ever got here. Why else do you suppose he signed up to go to Afghanistan at the last minute? He probably could not get a job in Seoul. They must know all about him there."

Tuesday, Krishna came back from Kathmandu. I saw Krishna myself later that day on the Guest House pathway, and asked if he knew what was happening on the surgery team. He told me he had heard all about it. He would deal with this problem. Park was re-assigned the very day that Krishna returned. Park's new job was in the outpatient clinic. Park would not be allowed to do any surgery or to scrub in. Park still joined the surgical team on ward rounds but was now in the back row. He spoke to nobody, looked at nobody, and shambled along like he was wearing shackles on his feet. The change in the way he acted was dramatic. The soft spoken and gentle Nepali surgeon, who had been Mark's second-in-command, was now the leader.

At one point during the next few days, Ellie came down to the Medical Ward where I was, to see the snakebite victim. He only owned three shirts, and that day he wore the blue one. A Maori whalebone ivory fishhook dangled from a black string around his neck as usual.

"Ellie, would you step into my office, please?" and we went out to the corridor for a second. He smiled. A quick glance confirmed that there was nobody else in earshot. "Have you, or anyone here, considered that Park might be a suicide risk?"

Ellie listened attentively and made a gesture with his cheeks as if he was sucking on a sourball. He squinted his eyes in a pained expression, as if he had not considered this. He finally said, "I see your point."

"Hey, I hope I am wrong but I'm just saying we have to think of all the angles. Ellie, I think Park is an outcast right now. He brought it on himself, that's for sure. But look, he has no manhood left. What would you do if you were him?"

"Well, Joe, I do not know what will happen here." He paused, searching for words. "But there is not much we can do." Another pause. "I suppose we owe it to the people at his NGO to see that he gets back safely."

"Yes, send him back.... but alive. He should not be our burden." He thanked me and we returned to the room where the snakebite victim lay in a semi-conscious state.

That evening we spent part of the time at the Guest House dinner table dissecting the dynamics of the surgical team just as if we had a scalpel. Al shook his head as he gave his opinion. "Not enough cutting time. Just not enough life experience." His eyebrows were raised as he spoke. He gestured with his fork. "The key element is that he could not deliver when it came time to do surgery. There is no forgiveness whatsoever for lack of technical competence." We all nodded in agreement as we ate.

Ellie told us that later in the week Park would return Seoul, spend two weeks there, and then go on to Afghanistan as originally planned. *God help the people in Kabul.* Park came to me to return the book I had lent him.

"I want to thank you for your kindness. I have not found the people here to be very friendly." I wondered whether that was truly what he thought, or whether it was just a way to avoid confronting his own shortcomings. *I just wanted him to go away.*

I was spending most of my time on Medical with our snakebite victim, but I went over to Surgical a few times to say hello to my student group and to Arupa the faculty member there. Life was subdued on Surgical, because you could not go into the Surgical Critical Ward without seeing the man Park had butchered struggling to breathe and dripping with sweat, while his wife stood silently by. She wore a blood-red *sari* and red bangles.

The patient continued to deteriorate for the next few days. When he was called to finish the surgery, Mark placed two drains, plastic tubes, in the abdomen to prevent the pancreatic juice from digesting the man's intestines, and these were now draining a foul liquid in to a collection bag. The patient's color was ashen. He ran a continuous fever. His incision was coming apart and there were several places where liquid stool seemed to be running out. Now the oldest son joined the patient's wife in the vigil. The smell of acrid stool permeated the room, with the added sweet smell of partly digested blood. We could not collect the drainage fast enough, and we needed to change the pads on his incision every hour or so. You could see the nurses gritting their teeth each time they went into the room. I admired their discipline and work ethic. The team discussed whether to operate again, but none of the surgeons thought that it would be helpful.

Wednesday was the usual medical education day, and the hour-long toot for the doctors on this day had been reserved for Park when he arrived. It was the custom to give each visiting doctor a time in the medical education schedule to present a topic of interest, and Park was still scheduled. Maybe it would provide Park a chance to redeem himself in some small way. Park chose to discuss IV fluids. He told me the topic the day before and I said, "Good. I hope you will get them to be more aggressive in what they order around here. From what I have seen, we do not use nearly as much IV fluid as they would in the US." He gave me a funny look.

I did not go to the toot. Al and Padma told me the story at dinner, from which Park was again absent. *Where does he eat?* I wondered. The report was, Park presented an argument to say that we should not be using IV fluids at all – the exact opposite of what I would have expected. The audience of doctors was incredulous. On questioning, Park produced the one article from the medical literature that served as the basis for his toot. It was something he read in a journal of experimental physiology which relied on mice. The other surgeons took strong exception to the premise during the discussion that followed, and Park was roundly embarrassed yet again.

As we discussed this, Dr. Cooper came in late from surgery. We passed his plate around to fill it, and told him about the discussion. He said he felt compelled to stand up and interrupt Park, because of all the misinformation. "Bloody fool," he added, "simply too junior a man to be doing this job." We asked if Cooper knew why Park was not eating with us. Somewhere along the way Cooper had learned that Park only ate one meal a day because he was concerned about gaining weight. I would have estimated Park's weight to be about one-hundred-sixty pounds.

The snakebite episode came to an end and I returned to Surgical in time to witness the morning of Park's last day at Tansen. We now had Hom, a short-term surgeon from the UK. Hom was from Delhi originally and had been in Nepal before. He stood with the team and with Park at the foot of the bed. The patient now had a rigid abdomen and terrible hip and shoulder pain. Hom's first question to Park was, "How did you get involved? Are you a surgeon?"

One of the Nepalis said, "No, he's more interested in theoretical physiology." I thought I detected a smirk as he said it. *One more dagger to Park's heart.* The wife seemed to be trying to read everyone's expression.

Park looked at Hom and said: "I did some inappropriate surgery, and then I panicked and did some unnecessary dissection."

Park took off his glasses and wiped his eyes, and started to cry. Park then apologized in English, "I am so sorry for the way this turned out. I wish I could have done better." *More to himself than to anybody*, I thought.

I wanted to avert my eyes; at first I looked at the others who were all trying to avoid eye contact as well. I looked around at the other patients in the room and it hit me that none of them had any personal stuff with them, the way an American patient would. No toiletries, no cards, no flowers. I was simultaneously listening/not listening as Park spoke. *Was he truly sorry for the pain he had caused? Or was it the blow to his ego? Had he learned anything? Anything at all?* While Park spoke, Hom looked at the graphic chart with a frown. Park left after that, and the team continued with the work at hand. Later that day, Hom brought the patient to Theater for repeat exploratory surgery. As they expected there was little they could do to repair what Park had done. All the suture lines were eroded by pancreatic fluid. The patient died the day after Park left for Seoul. I was not around for that event.

In the afternoon I went Flat Street, to the internet café. Sloppy yellow paint job on the woodwork had been splashed onto the plate glass window. Next door was a store that sold TVs and refrigerators. The boy at the counter gestured for me to sit at the computer closest to the door. About twenty feet away, Magar women smoked hand-rolled *cheroots* while they squatted next to their vegetables which were displayed on a blanket on the ground. The blue tractor went by, laying down a trail of blue diesel fumes, and the smell of smoke wafted through from somewhere somebody was preparing corn on the cob over charcoal. I could see a cow on the far end of Flat Street.

Today the internet was working. I checked my email. There was a message from Celeste, asking about my spiritual journey, hoping that I was growing my horizons, and asking if I felt much different now that I was settling in.

I sat at the internet café reading the message. I read it again. *What journey? What horizons? You have got to be kidding.* I started to write the story of Park, the story of the snakebite, the children who had died, the guy whose vomit got on my knees, everything.

Then stopped.

I can't even describe this. I found the delete key and held my finger over it for a second as I reread what I had just wrote.

Deleted it all.

Started over from a blank page. Sent a short reply to say: *It was busy here and I was too shell shocked to know the answer to any of those questions.*

Sandy's Report From Mugu

Every two years UMN sends a team to Mugu for two weeks to provide medical care there. There are two ways to get to Mugu. The first is to walk, for a week or more. The second is to land at the airstrip on the mountainside above the town, then hike down a steep hill for about an hour. The airstrip was built back in the days when the American CIA was working with the Nepali government to spy on the Chinese from places on the border, and Mugu is at about eleven-thousand feet in the Himalayas. The people there are considered to be among the poorest in Asia.

The medical team in 2007 was on an expedition in the truest sense of the word. They needed to bring in one hundred percent of their supplies, including all the food they planned to eat. They reviewed their boxes, as well as the list of equipment, many times to make sure they brought what they needed. One of the photos showed row upon row of numbered boxes laid out to be loaded onto the plane at the Kathmandu airport. At each end of the airstrip in Mugu is a precipitous drop off, hence no second chance at landing or taking off. Perfect visibility was needed because there was no landing tower. *It took guts just to get in the plane.* When they landed, the team carried all their supplies a mile downhill to the village below and walked back up for more. At that elevation, a walk like this makes your legs burn and you must pause to breathe every few steps, even without carrying cargo on your back.

The team sterilized the surgical instruments with a pressure cooker such as you might use in your kitchen, heated with a small gas stove. In the morning and afternoon the same pressure cooker also boiled the water for tea. At that elevation, water boils at a lower temperature. The team "camped out" for the duration in an unused building. There was no electricity. The "clinic" had not been used for a while and the walls were grimy. The team was careful about all those boxes, because items can still get lost unless there is a system for where to pile them and which ones to open. It was a tribute to their planning that the team set up shop and used their skills. Though the women were poor, the local costume included gold earrings that were so heavy the wearer also would use an extra loop of leather thong over the ear to hold them on. *It is a pity they can't eat the gold.*

You might think this mission to Mugu was glamorous, because after all it is a sort of a backpacking trip with surgery thrown in. *Possibly the ultimate way to trek.* After the first such trip you would never think that way again. Two weeks is a long time to go without hot water or plumbing if you are not used to it and the fun disappears quickly when your patient is suffering. "Hard core" is a better term. Not just anybody can be on the team. It is chosen from among longterm volunteers and missionaries. Mission Hospital contributed one person, a doctor named Sandy, who was London-trained like her husband. She joined others from throughout UMN.

Everyone in the town stood patiently in line for a medical exam, so that the team could sort out the various illnesses types and devise a plan of surgery over the coming days. At first they were surprised that all the women of the Mugu region seemed so young. Then they realized that the situation was a bit more complicated – what was really happening was that all the women over the age of thirty-nine had developed one illness or another and died. *Women flat-out died when they reached menopause.* Sandy was about thirty-four herself. It took the medical team a bit of time to realize who was missing in the balance of age groups. Once they grasped this, they had some sleepless nights, and Sandy was in tears as she described it to us.

The team was shocked to learn that it was the practice in Mugu not to feed a newborn baby until the third day of life, "To see if it was strong enough to live." Sandy reported that during the whole two weeks, there was not one occasion in which a woman of Mugu smiled or laughed. Life was grim at eleven-thousand feet in the Himalayas.

When the lights came back on in the room, everyone sat there quietly for a moment. Sandy said she thought that Tansen was wonderful compared to what it was like in Mugu.

Photo facing page: The wall display of snakes in the E.R. The four main kinds of poisonous snakes in our area.

The Messenger of Shiva

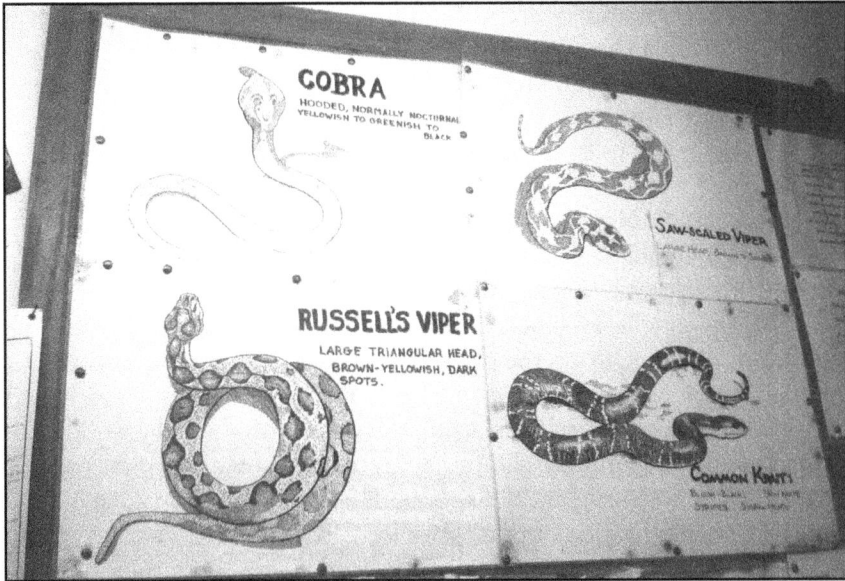

There are no snakes in Hawaii where I live. Before the trip I found two medical websites on snakebite treatment in Nepal. There are seventy-six varieties of snakes in Nepal, and more than two-dozen are poisonous. It's a problem.

Some snake venoms cause coagulopathy, a condition that prevents the blood from clotting; others cause paralysis, and the victim dies of strangulation because their breathing muscles no longer work. A third main category is the kind that causes a nasty bite wound that is very painful and gets infected. Venom from the King Cobra contains aspects of all three. The outcome after a bite depends on the amount of venom, the location of the bite, and the size of the victim. A small child bitten on the face will die more rapidly and surely than an adult bitten on the leg or bitten with a glancing strike. There are no snakes in the Himalayas – it's too cold there.

A person bitten out in the countryside, who dies before getting to the hospital, will not be captured in the statistics. Bites by a non-poisonous snake – do they count as a "real" bite? What if the victim is not sure which kind it was? These are the kind of issues that get in the way of making a clear clean epidemiological pronouncement on snakebite as a public health issue. Also, the Nepali doctors tend to rely on medical studies from centers in India, which has a different grouping of wild snakes than Nepal. The antivenin (also known as the antidote) for snakebite in Nepal is made in Kathmandu and is free of charge to all hospitals and health centers, but there have been few studies on the correct dose of the antivenin, or the timing of the dose. One antivenin is made to a formula that encompasses all the possible snakes – how does that impact the dose for a known specific snake? A doctor needs to guess the answer to these questions.

Tansen is in the hills, but overlooks a large valley, and many of our patients came from the *Terai*, up the winding road from Butwal. The main food crop of Nepal is rice, grown in flooded paddies. The paddies are separated by dikes, and there are many locations where the paddies have been carved out of steep hillsides. Before the monsoon, the fields lay bare, vast stretches of cracked dirt with a mosaic of dikes between, awaiting moisture. During the dry season, the snakes can live anywhere.

When the rain comes the people begin the ancient steps of working a rice paddy – the nursery beds; using the water buffalo and a wooden plow to prepare the muddy paddy; the teams of women in bright red *saris*, bent over to transplant the shoots. The colorful *saris* make it easy to spot the workers. From a distance they look like to be red dots, far away.

In early June the torrential rains start. In the *Terai*, with the summer temperature hovering around a hundred and ten degrees, the coming of Monsoon forces the snakes to move. Since the only high dry ground is where the local farmers live, each farmer's house becomes a sort of Noah's Ark – the place where all the farm creatures go – water buffalo, goats, and chickens – and during monsoon, snakes. *Did Noah bring snakes on the Ark?*

Everybody seemed to know somebody who died from snakebite, and one day during my language lesson, my Nepali language tutor told me of a five-year-old niece who died this way. In Hindu lore, a snake is a messenger from Shiva, the destroyer; Shiva uses snakes to summon people. There is a fatalism associated with snakebite.

At Mission Hospital a patient with a snakebite story is automatically admitted overnight. The staff is well schooled on antivenin administration and the response is efficient. The Emergency Room is run on "the Australian Model," and patients admitted from there are quickly moved to the in-patient wards for treatment. The ER is really just one sixteen-by-sixteen foot room that is deceptively small for a hospital that sees one-hundred-thousand outpatient visits a year and serves five-hundred-thousand people in its catchment area.

I laughed out loud when I first saw the high shelf in the Emergency Room. There were about a dozen pickled snakes in jars, trophies of previous skirmishes with the Messenger of Shiva. Most had labels made of the old-fashioned sticky cloth medical tape, a kind they no longer use

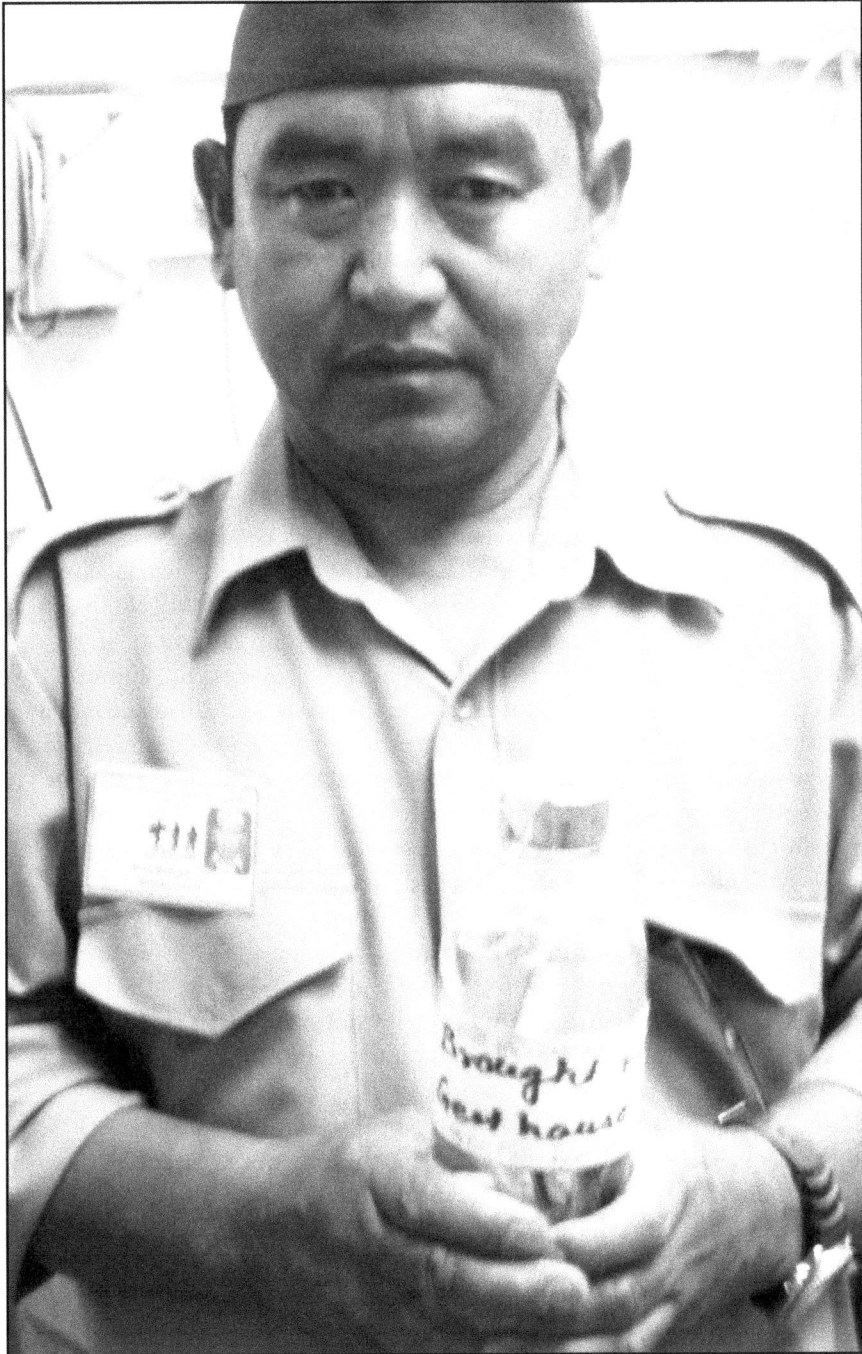

One of the *Chowkidars*, showing me a jar from the high shelf in the ER, containing a pickled snake.

in the US, with a handwritten note as to the acquisition of the specimen inside. The *Chowkidar*, a security guard in a crisp khaki uniform with black *topi*, climbed on a stool and got them down from the shelf for me to examine. A sad one: "This krait bit a five-year-old boy on the face and he died." The next one was: "Brought from Guest House Apartment Number 3." In the jar was a Krait, with venom sixteen times more deadly than cobra venom. I was renting Guest House Number 5 for the summer and was just beginning to feel comfortable there. The *Chowkidar* and the rest of the staff all watched as I read the label. "Sometimes the formaldehyde gets milky and we throw them out. Every year we replenish the display. We use these to help the victim identify the kind of snake that bit them."

The snake population of the Guest House complex was decimated a few years back when a Scandinavian Missionary Doctor lived there and made it a personal crusade to drive all the snakes from the neighborhood, a veritable modern day Saint Patrick. We were in a lull from which the local snakes had not yet recovered. Since the snakes only bite when provoked, many of the local population do not kill them as our Swedish Missionary had done. "If you keep your garbage clear, there will be fewer mice and if there are fewer mice the snakes will stay away." *Keep the garbage clear.* In apartment three, the snake had slithered in via the shower drain. Always *leave a dish over the drain when not is use. Also use the flashlight at night, even when only going from the bedroom to the bathroom.*

About two weeks after I arrived in Tansen, the usual Wednesday mid-morning toot was set aside for the subject of snakebite response. Llewellyn "Ellie" Jones was the Aussie doctor in charge of medical education. Ellie had a toothy smile and a twinkle in his eye which imparted an element of fun and intrigue. "You'll want to come to this Joe, it will put your mind at ease," he said as he invited me. Mind was pronounced "moind" and I found myself mulling over the word.

As I entered the conference room, I looked around at the other attendees – about ten foreign missionary doctors and more than a dozen Nepali interns, residents and medical students. I found a seat in the back. The tutorial was given by another missionary doctor from Oz, named Will Masters. Will is tall and athletic with a boyish outlook. He shared the Adult Medical Service with his wife who is also an MD. There was a weekly Wednesday afternoon cricket session and Will usually bowled. "I'm Australian, it's in my blood."

The toot was a scholarly review of available literature including laying out the questions related to the dose of antivenin. In Tansen we were mainly worried about Kraits and the King Cobra. Will ended with a short discussion of treatment and said, "We have a ventilator here but we have never used it. It would be ideal therapy for a victim of a paralytic snakebite, because these patients would survive with excellent results if we could get them through the short-term paralytic phase."

Of all the people in the room, a show of hands indicated that only Will, Ellie, and I had previously used a mechanical ventilator. After the meeting I volunteered to look at the problem. "I have used these machines since nineteen-seventy-eight in the US. Give me the keys. I want to take it out for a spin."

Samuel was the driving force to acquire the ventilators, which is why the ventilator and supplies were locked in a nondescript closet on the Pediatric Ward. A few days later we met there and Samuel got out the key as he spoke.

"We have used a mechanical ventilator only one time, on a patient who was hit by a car and had a head injury. He had a remarkable recovery after craniotomy here, but died of ventilator-acquired pneumonia. We aren't sure why. We did realize that in the US or UK or Australia when we write ventilator orders, it's really up to the skill of the nursing staff to carry them out and we doctors don't know exactly what nurses do to make the difference."

My response was, "*Thik Cha.* Let's take a look at the machine."

We opened the big gray steel cabinet and out tumbled a pile of stuff. There were actually three mechanical ventilators. What followed was the kind of scene you might expect at a classic car rally. It was the medical equivalent of two guys looking under the hood of a recently-restored '57 Chevy, gawking at the primitiveness on the one hand; appreciating the mechanical elegance; and talking about the thought process behind the way the engine was rebuilt. *How can we make this thing run?*

Samuel's stash included two different models of ventilator. First was the "little yellow Aussie bush box" which did not even use electricity – it cycled using only the pressure of the oxygen tank to which it was attached. It was sleek and cute but had a drawback: it could only deliver 100% oxygen, and was not able to mix in any room air.

The next machine was a "Puritan-Bennett LP 6" transport ventilator. We settled on it as our first choice. It was simple, just four main controls and some alarms. Using duck tape, we could rig it to boost the oxygen percent. I told Samuel my friends back in Maine would get a kick out of learning one more use for duck tape.

We attached the tubing and turned it on to inflate the little black rubber test bag, which also had little patches of duck tape to seal the holes. *Oh yeah...* The machine chugged while we had an old-fashioned bull session, fiddling with the dials and alarms as if we were adjusting a carburetor. As potential clinical partners, we needed a sense of how we would work together on this. We bounced ideas around and it seemed to click. Samuel was very practical in his approach to the problems we would inevitably face. I was reminded of times I helped my dad work on one home repair project or another when I was in high school.

I told Samuel I could mentally picture the exact layout of the dials on the old Bear One ventilator and could draw from memory the documentation flowchart we used to use.

He said, "When I used to be a flight instructor, I would ask the students to draw the instrument panel from memory. You are doing the same thing with this. Good."

"Samuel, I am totally into it. If we use this vent and you *don't* let me in on it, I will be pissed." He winced a bit. Samuel never used bad language.

We owned ten sets of tubing, and there was an inline device, like a sponge, to humidify the gas we delivered. We listed what we did not have: no continuous cardiac monitor; no Arterial Blood Gas machine, no respirometer, no way to accurately measure the oxygen, no ability to measure the Negative Inspiratory Force (NIF). We could not deliver PEEP with this thing.

Clinical success would be determined by seeing that the tube was in place, whether the chest seemed to be going up and down, what the pulse and blood pressure were doing, and what the pulse oximetry reading was. No "minute volume," no "compliance," no "wedge pressure." We would be flying through clouds in the Sopwith Camel of mechanical ventilators. I wondered what my dad would think if he heard me now. *This is just the kind of project Stan would tackle. He was always trying to do something for which a normal person would hire a professional. He would attempt to jury rig anything. Now, I am trying to do something ambitious with about half the tools I need. Just like Stan. Somehow he usually managed to pull it off. I wonder if we will.*

"If worse comes to worse, and something goes wrong, we just unhook the machine and use a manual ventilator instead," which meant we would be ambu-bagging, possibly for hours or days. To use an ambu-bag was the way they did it now; the beauty of having a ventilator is to free the staff from doing this chore.

We put all the equipment back in the closet and I took the Manufacturer's Manual back to the Guest House with me. Over the next two weeks, I used a computer in the hospital library to write a policy and procedure that adapted the machine to our purposes. By this time I was busy during the day supervising students in Clinical, so I puttered around with the policy in the evenings. It seemed like the junior doctors were always using the library computer for medical searches, so I had to try to find a time when it was available. There was not any sense of urgency.

On June eighth there was a torrential downpour and we thought, "Monsoon has come." After weeks of stifling heat and humidity, there was palpable joy. As the rain came in torrents there was shouting and singing as the local Nepalis literally danced in the street in the rain. Rows of pots and pans appeared under the drip line of every house – women could now get water without a daily trip to the well down the street! But the next day was dry and the heat built up again. Monsoon would be late. The temperature simmered at about a hundred degrees Fahrenheit each day.

The following Wednesday there was a special toot just for the nurses. It was devoted to the subject of Pediatric Life Support. A major component of successful resuscitation is being able to insert and care for an endotracheal tube, a device inserted through the mouth and into the lungs. Ambhika and all the senior nurses – the "Sisters" – were there.

You would not expect to find an intubation manikin from the Laerdal Company in rural Nepal, but we owned one, brought by another short-term visitor to Mission Hospital. Lily Johnson was a nurse from the Midwest who was friends with Samuel and his wife Trina. Lily was the daughter of missionaries. She knew that she should not come empty handed for a visit to a mission outpost. When Lily planned her trip, she asked Samuel what she could bring, and her church contributed the money to buy it. Then Lily brought it as personal baggage to rural Nepal. The nurses practiced with it and we took photos for her to show the folks back home. Doctors and nurses in rural Nepal also had the latest videos and computer simulations from the American Heart Association.

I finished writing the policy on a Saturday before church, using the library computer before anybody else. The sermon that day was about accepting sacrifices for your faith and dealing with persecution. Evidently there had been a recent incident in a neighboring village in which some young Hindus attacked a Nepali Christian man who was now in the hospital. They beat him with bamboo sticks, fracturing his ribs and jaw. This was a very unusual act of religious intolerance from what I had seen. Nepali people were actually very mellow. The man was planning to return to his village and report the attackers. The sermon was designed to reinforce the resolve of the congregation to stay on the Christian path.

After church I went for a walk to the *Bajar* and checked my email. It was not working, so I walked through some different parts of town than usual. I found out where the movie theater was located. Walking nearby I heard music and laughter coming from behind the curtain of an open door and peeked inside to find fifteen couples who were enthusiastically participating in a Bhangra dance class. I got back to the hospital compound in time for English-language service at the Guest House.

The next week started off with stifling heat, Sunday at change-of-shift report I was already sweating at seven in the morning. Monday I arrived on the Surgical Ward, planning to spend the day supervising first-year students there. Arupa, another faculty member, was also there with a group of third-year students.

Thus far there had been a leisurely quality to the ventilator project, like being on a jet taxiing out to the runway. At eight-thirty Monday morning there was a sudden change, as if we were gathering speed for takeoff. Will Masters came by to tell me I should go to the ER. Samuel was with a snakebite victim. I gave Arupa a hurried farewell and rushed off.

The victim was twenty-two-years old, twitching on the ER stretcher. Pulse one-hundred-sixty beats per minute, blood pressure two-hundred over one-hundred-forty and cyanotic. An IV had been started and we were ventilating with an ambu-bag, setting up for intubation. Samuel guided Surendra, one of the Nepali doctors, as Surendra used the laryngoscope and ET tube. With a sense of relief we confirmed that the tube was in the trachea. The patient had ten milligrams of valium on board. We pumped the bag and his cyanosis abated – he "pinked up."

Surendra stepped out and returned with the two men who brought the patient to the hospital, a brother and a brother-in-law. He asked them what happened. They were excited and spoke in a stream of Nepali so fast I could not understand a single word. The patient's name was Dharsha; he was from the Parbas valley about ten miles away. He'd gotten up at three o'clock in the morning to urinate, then came back saying he'd been bitten on the hand. At first his brother took him to Lumbini Medical Center (LMC) which was not far from his house in Parbas. This was a small hospital that was trying to start up in competition with Mission Hospital but didn't have many patients. At LMC the doctors did not recognize the seriousness at first since there was no visible bite mark. LMC did not have any antivenin in any case and just gave him antihistamines. As Dharsha continued to get worse his brothers pulled him out of LMC and brought him to Mission Hospital in a taxi. Surendra took one look at him and decided to pull out the stops.

Once the tube was in and taped, Samuel went to get the equipment while I bagged Dharsha. Six of us moved him to an in-patient area. Our destination was the Medical Critical Ward, a four bed room close to the nurse's station. The trip included going down a steep ramp while bagging the patient, oxygen tank trailing behind. We made a clatter as we moved. As we got to the room, the charge nurse told me that two beds were empty and one was occupied by a twenty-two-year-old diabetic in renal failure.

We hooked him up to the ventilator. *Chest going up and down. Hot damn, this is slick*, I thought to myself. Dharsha got a round of antivenin, ten vials. No effect. Foley catheter, restraints. Re-taped the tube and repeated the x-ray. Obviously he'd already been envenomated, which meant the antivenin was too late. *He was going to stay paralyzed until the poison wore off.*

Will came by and said it must have been a Krait. "Nocturnal, small snake, hardly any visible bite, mainly paralytic. Look at his eyes."

Sure enough, Dharsha had "Doll's Eyes," a peculiar telltale sign. *The damnedest thing.* "The literature says that the twelve cranial nerves are particularly affected and he may have double vision for six months after this if he survives." The name of the snake is not pronounced the way it is spelled; the Nepalis have a way to roll the "r" so it is more like "Krrrrrait," onomatopoeia to evoke the faint sound of a snake's tongue. "The fangs do not leave more than a pinprick sometimes. The literature says he will be paralyzed for two days on average."

Will decided to administer another round of antivenin and a neostigmine challenge. The neostigmine did not reverse the paralysis but it seemed to cause an immediate rise in pulse to one-hundred-seventy and blood pressure to one-ninety over one-ten along with a drop in pulse oximetry. We feverishly rechecked everything to make sure it was all working. We thought he was about to crash. *It will be over before it started.*

Dharsha also had a ventricular heave, a sign that the heart muscle was struggling. "Cardiotoxicity is part of it. If his heart muscle is paralyzed there is nothing we can do and he will die." We decided to ride out the change in vital signs. At that time the Hospital Chaplain came by. He is a young man about thirty with a charismatic smile. We knelt at the head of the bed and said Christian prayers for Dharsha. *Will this work on a Hindu? There is not much else to try. I really wanted to win this one.* Curiously, Dharsha settled down a bit. It occurred to me that *all the prayer at Mission Hospital was not simply going-through-the-motions. We needed those prayers.*

After we stabilized Dharsha, we sketched out a routine for his care. Nurses were re-assigned and I was to be available to troubleshoot. We arranged to teach the junior medical staff and the nurses about the machine. We kept the patient sedated. His brothers were around, and I got the opportunity to talk with them for the first time. One brother spoke a bit of English. He was in a daze, "I don't know what to do. They tell us all these things and it seems so strange. I have never seen anything like this."

Dharsha was twenty-two-years old and had been working as a cook in India but had returned home three months earlier. They were rice farmers and I later learned that they still used water buffalo in their paddies and fields. Their house had no electricity. A rain in the valley had filled their paddies. The snake had been around the house for a few days but they did not want to kill it, just drive it away. It kept coming back, they said.

I told them to kill the damn thing.

In Nepal, people conduct all aspects of their life in public, and this is true even in the hospital. There is always a crowd of onlookers no matter what is happening. So at first we thought nothing of the stream of people that popped their head into the room, some even asking questions. The word spread of what we had done and what had happened to Dharsha, and it seemed that every employee popped their head in. Total strangers were coming by and we started trying to limit the number of curious onlookers. Later that day, a crowd of men gathered near the room, as the young girl with renal failure died. She was not a candidate for resuscitation. There were about a dozen men, waiting quietly as her death added to the drama. Her body lay behind the drapes for an hour until the doctor wrote the death certificate and the men lifted it onto the stretcher.

While Dharsha stabilized, I started a series of small toots. For each group of three or four doctors and nurses I went over the machine, the assessments, the dials, answered all questions. I talked with them about "phasing in," which is a way to assess whether the machine and patient are working together. An experienced critical care nurse develops a sixth sense about "phasing in" and uses it to guide decisions about how much sedation to use. I encouraged Dharsha's brothers to speak in his ear and re-assure him. The Nepalis were self-conscious about it, but gave Dharsha words of encouragement and re-assurance.

This was just the first day; and we did not know how long Dharsha would be on the ventilator. I eventually went home for dinner, but only after I left the phone number to my apartment on a paper taped to the wall. At dinner Al told us that his dad was a GP and his mum was an anesthesiologist in the UK, and every evening they used to talk medicine at the dinner table. Al loved it when the story of the patient was told as a living breathing story apart from the scientific facts of disease, which were boring. As he spoke I could picture him as an inquisitive ten-year-old boy, listening eagerly for what's next. *No wonder he's such a storyteller.* I told him I had no idea how this one would turn out, we would have to wait and see. Then we talked about Tibet. He was planning to go there for a month after Tansen when his girlfriend came. He would not tell us anything about her, other than her name, "Miss Boston."

I said, "Doesn't she have a first name?"

"Miss Boston to you. Just leave it at that."

At eleven o'clock I was awakened by a phone call from the night intern. Nobody ever called my phone at the apartment, so I was startled at first. I got my clothes on quickly, buttoning my shirt as I walked the hundred meters to the Medical Ward, adjusting the *topi* just so. With my torch I watched for snakes on the stone path as I walked. When I got there, the intern, the nurse, and the nursing students were all huddling around the machine. Dharsha was doing as well as could be expected, that was not the problem. In fact, he looked clean and comfortable, the same way that American nurses would have cared for him.

We turned to the machine, which was running on battery. There was something wrong with the electrical supply. Three of us got on our hands and knees to look closely at the setup and trace it from the wall. Turns out that the wall socket was 220 volts, and the current was running through two metal boxes with dials on them and transformers inside, to convert it to 110 because it was an American machine. *They don't talk about this kind of offbeat electrical problem in nursing school.* Again I was transported back to rewiring the house in Maine with my dad. *What would Stan do if he was here?* For some reason, one box had stopped working. It was hot to the touch. *Glad it didn't catch fire.* Ellie came, and I was surprised to see him in glasses, not contacts. None of us could get it going; there were no bright ideas. Ellie pronounced the word "broight." There probably was a sensor that would not reset until the box cooled down. The biomedical engineer was away. We could not fix it so we prepared to ambu-bag Dharsha overnight. I could sense that the others were looking at me so I tried to be optimistic. Soon, the machine breathed its last as the battery died. *Stan would just turn the no-damn-good thing off. He is a realist.* And so, we switched to bagging. We were going to bag until morning. *Let's see – twenty breaths a minute, sixty minutes per hour, eight hours... that's nine thousand six hundred breaths.* It was going to be a long night, especially since the staff nurses still had twenty-seven other patients to look after.

There are few activities as boring as ambu-bagging a patient for hours at a time. Observe the patient's effort, and each time the person seems to breathe in, squeeze the bag with both hands. I assigned twenty-minute shifts, and we took turns. I taught the students how to phase in, timing each delivered breath with the patient's efforts. We all talked to pass the time. I learned that one of the nursing students was a member of the Sherpa tribe, the group that serves as porters to Mount Everest. To visit her family required a five-day trip from Tansen, the last two days on foot. I told them about the hospitals in Hawaii and the equipment in the US. They were curious about my daughters. I wished I had a picture with me.

One brother slept on a bedroll under the bed, while the other closed his eyes, slouching in a recliner. By this time I was used to relatives who camped out – it was the way things were done. I did not bat an eyelash.

The brothers seemed restless and finally they said, "Let us help."

Sure why not. I showed them how to use the ambu-bag, and they each took turns with the twenty-minute shifts. I got my camera and took pictures of one brother as he bagged. He smiled as he pumped away. I summoned the student nurses from other parts of the building and showed them how to use the ambu-bag. Then we got the *Chowkidar* with his fistful of antique-looking keys, and told him to take the students and scour the hospital compound for a box like the one that had cut out. I offered a hundred rupees to the person who found a box that would substitute.

An hour later they returned in a small procession, carrying some odd electrical boxes but none was the kind we needed, so there was no winner in this impromptu contest. At seven in the morning, we discovered that the box had cooled off. I plugged it in. *It did not catch fire, a good sign.* It seemed to work, so we fired up the machine. I decided to stay awake and see if Dharsha would improve that day. *After all, the venom was bound to wear off.* I put my palm on his chest and noted that his heave had gone away, indicating his heart muscle was better.

At seven-thirty there was always a medical staff briefing in the conference room. Each day, this was accompanied by prayer and bible readings. I did not usually go, but that morning I walked up the steps and sat on the bench with the night intern. When the night intern gave report on Dharsha's condition, Norma, the pediatrician, stood up.

"I believe that God sent Joe Niemczura to us to help with this patient. I just want to lift Joe up to the Lord."

I was a bit startled by that remark. This was a thought that had not occurred to me. *We were getting off into some kind of new zone, a place I had not been before.* I was speechless.

Tuesday was Day Two and we decided we would try to wean Dharsha from the machine. Our strategy was to put him on SIMV mode and dial down the machine breaths. The doctor covering the Medical service was pushing the idea that we wean him but I stood my ground and said that I knew every set of weaning criteria published in the last thirty years and Dharsha met none of them. "He will just plain die if we extubate him now." Ellie came by and we engaged in an erudite discussion as to how one might assess the return of breathing after this kind of paralysis. "Do you suppose the degree of paralysis can be quantified and used to predict weanability?" Neither of us knew the answer to that one. The question was stated in a bantering tone to imply that we both knew we were suffering from delusions of grandeur. *Certainly there is relevant physiology to guide us, but I don't know what it may be. I wonder if Ellie is bullshitting as much as I am right now.* We looked at his "Doll's Eyes" again, bobbling Dharsha's head almost absentmindedly from side-to-side to elicit the sign. *Maybe we were hoping that the tenth time we looked for them, he would no longer have Doll's Eyes.*

Ellie disappeared without telling me where he was going, but a half hour later he returned with the "chain of four" stimulator from the Operating Theater. He triumphantly announced that we *could* quantify the paralysis with this machine; after all it was what the Theater staff used during postoperative recovery. At first the way he pronounced it, the word came out like "*China Fawe*" and I did not know what he was talking about.

"Speak English" I said.
"I am speaking the King's English, thank you," he replied.
"That can't be true. The Nepalis speak the King's English. I can understand them perfectly. I studied Nepali for seven months. I didn't know I would need to study Auzzie 'til I got here."

He squinted at me with one eye and changed topics. "Just watch this and you will learn something." He sat down at the bedside and tested the "chain of four" device, first on himself, then on Dharsha. Results were inconclusive. We got no useful information from it. He looked at me with a rueful grin. I told him, "Ellie, it was a great idea and I wished I had thought of it." *So much for science. We were dealing with the Messenger of Shiva here.*

This was still Tuesday, Dharsha's second day on the machine. We arranged a longer toot for the whole junior staff, about a dozen doctors crowded around the bed. For this I gave a lecture in English and Surendra translated into Nepali. Surendra was considered to be among the brightest of the batch, and it was a test of his language ability to translate the medical jargon, which is a very specialized vocabulary. We decided to use two languages so as to make absolutely certain that all questions were answered, though this may have not been strictly necessary since all the junior doctors started off with pretty good English. This prompted a sort of game-within-a-game. The Nepali doctors could hear what I said, then hear how Surendra translated, and compare for themselves how they in turn would have translated if they were in Surendra's place, being put on the spot. When Surendra explained some of the difficult words or concepts, they were therefore able to enjoy it on several levels. Surendra solidified his reputation for intelligence and a sense of humor.

For me, this toot was a turning point. Up to this time, most of the medical staff did not know what exactly to do about me, where I might fit in the social hierarchy of this hospital. Men are not nurses in Nepal. I had been careful not to be too assertive for fear of seeming to criticize, so few knew that I had fifteen years of Intensive Care experience in the US. Until now, my high technology background had seemed totally irrelevant to a hospital with no defibrillator or heart monitor. I had not expected to be in the position to do this kind of teaching. Here I was, giving them some information they could use, showing some unexpected expertise, and the patient who had benefited from it was laying there in front of us. The nursing staff was also viewing me differently.

Sometimes a patient just wakes up and resumes breathing as if nothing had happened. This seemed to be taking awhile, and we were worried. After about three days, the patient is likely to develop ventilator-acquired pneumonia, which would be very difficult to treat. Our selection of antibiotics was limited and we would have trouble supplying the staff for a prolonged period of mechanical ventilation. I realized that I really wanted him to live. This was also not good. I knew I would cry when he died. *Bummer*. We switched from valium to morphine for sedation. Morphine would have a shorter half-life, and might make it easier to wean the guy.

The second night, the electricity cut out again. I made another walk to Medical, careful to wear my *topi*, though nobody even commented on it when I got there. This time the biomed guy was back in town. He came to the hospital and explained to us that during the night, there was less demand for current in the town of Tansen, which caused a voltage surge. It was inconvenient that the box was overheating, but without it, the surge would damage the equipment, which would be impossible to repair. He brought a different box and the problem was solved after only two hours of bagging.

Wednesday morning Ellie was in charge, and this time we decided to wean using a T-piece strategy. This is a small adapter that connects the one-inch diameter endotracheal tube, to an oxygen tube of a different size, with a short rebreather device on the end, shaped like the letter "T." "Do we have a T-piece in this town?" he asked.

"Good question. I have not seen one for sale at the *Bajar*. We should have sent to Kathmandu for one. Are you much of a whittler?" I think he could detect the sarcasm.

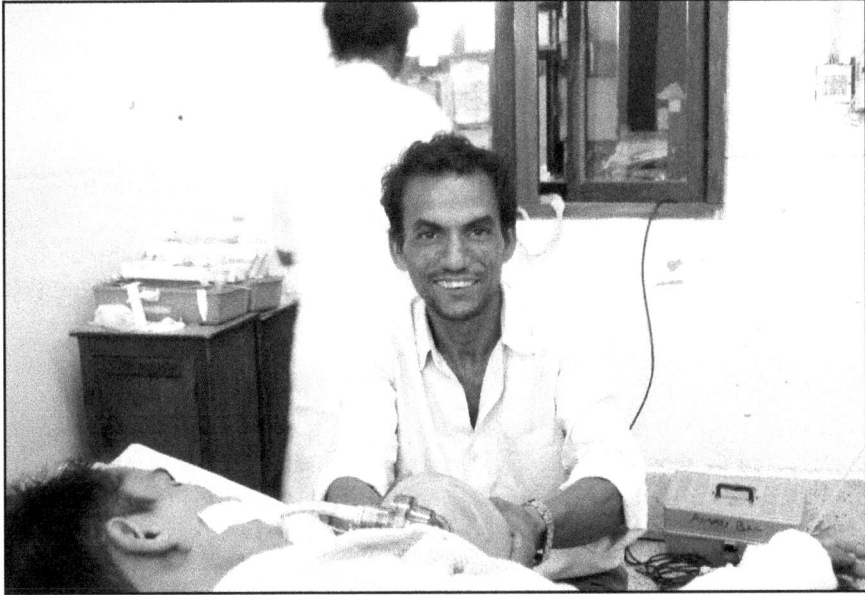

Dharsha's brother, using an ambu-bag at 0300, smiling for the camera. He was cheerful about bagging, because it felt like he was doing something for his brother instead of passively waiting.

"O ye of little faith!" His eyes twinkled. *Nothing fazes this guy.*

Ellie went to the nurse's station. On one side was a junk drawer like the one my mother had in her kitchen when I was growing up – odds and ends, a Tuborg beer can opener, a magnet, a small, sticky brown bottle of oil of peppermint, 3-in-1 oil from India, odd pieces of colored glass, and part of a broken stethoscope. He held up a three-inch diameter ring made of red rubber with talcum powder on it, and said, "I was looking for one of these last week." I didn't know what it was. He gleefully announced that it was a pessary, and slipped it into his pocket. Next were different sized screws, nuts and bolts – assorted hand tools. Ellie muttered as he used two hands to pull out the drawer and dump it on the counter. I could not make out what he was saying.

After a minute of rummaging he found a white plastic venturi adapter and held it up to the light, turning it back and forth. One end was an inch in diameter and the other would fit the oxygen hose. *Perfect.* He washed it in the sink and declared his intention to modify it into a T-piece using his jackknife and a bit of the old-fashioned sticky cloth tape. "A masterpiece of improvisation, if I do say so myself." Pronounced "*moyself*." I still had trouble with his English.

115

We brought it into the room and rigged it up for a trial of weaning with the T-piece. It seemed to go okay, from what we could tell – after two hours we thought it was a "decent interval on the T-piece" and we all agreed to pull the tube. Surendra came by, and we all posed for pictures with Dharsha, who was still in a daze but seemed to be breathing spontaneously. We suctioned him one last time and removed the tube. He was breathing on his own. He could not focus his eyes. *Doll's eyes.* He did not speak. He was using accessory muscles to breathe, which was worrisome. *Maybe his diaphragm was still paralyzed.* We put him on a rebreather and cranked up the oxygen.

Within an hour we realized that he still had no gag reflex whatsoever. *He was a sitting duck to aspirate his own secretions and die.* His temperature spiked to 102. We gave him paracetamol rectally. *Maybe this was a big mistake and we should have waited one more day.* I repositioned him on his side and did vigorous chest physiotherapy, using my hands to shake his secretions loose and improve his oxygen. I suctioned him using a special technique to put the catheter in the trachea "blind." He did cough up some mucus that way. Lastly, I did the only other thing I could think of, which was to reposition him flat on his stomach and put in an oral airway to keep him from choking. I taped it in place. He did not even gag on it.

Will came by and told me that if Dharsha arrested again he would not be reintubated. "We already expended a lot of resources on him. We all think you did a great job but he's got pneumonia now, and if it is bad enough to cause respiratory failure we can't keep him on the ventilator for weeks. Maybe it was not meant to be." Will was philosophical but after looking through the chart he decided to adjust the antibiotic and order more chest physiotherapy.

I felt tired. After Will left I went to the bedside. I put my hand on Dharsha's shoulder and spoke to him in English. "I want you to know that I tried as hard as I could. We all want the best for you. If you die today I want you to know that I am sorry to see you go." I had only been in Tansen four weeks but had seen more than fifteen deaths. *This was one more death. One more statistic.* Dharsha was floating off downstream, away from shore. Soon to be picked up by the current.

My mind was elsewhere at dinner. The big discussion was the toot that Park had given. The medical students at the Guest House then watched *Shakespeare in Love* for the eighth time. I went to bed early. *I felt like I was coming down from a speed run.* I contemplated the idea that I could put in long hours when I was younger but right now I preferred the day shift. That night I dreamed that I was at the Common Ground Fair in Maine, the organic farming festival, wandering among the tents.

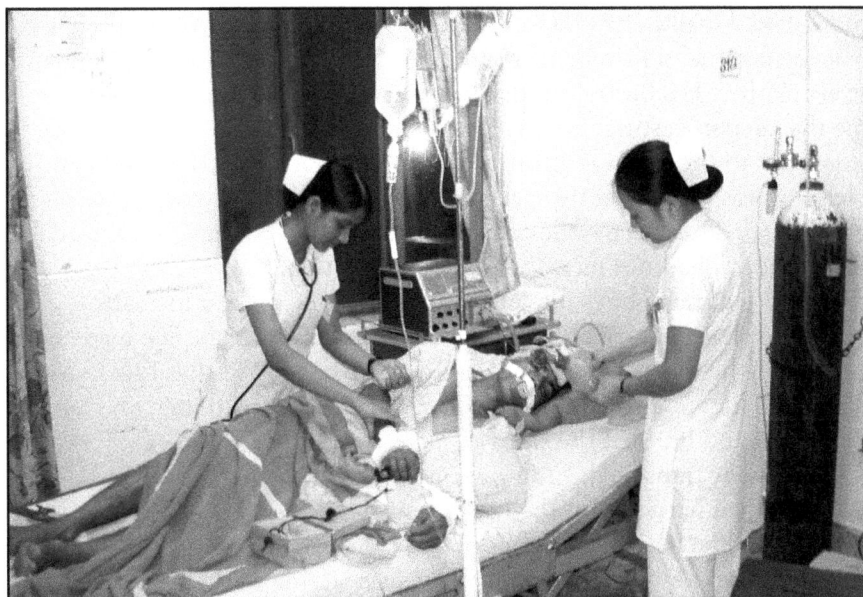

Two TNS students taking care of Dharsha during the night. He is being ambu-bagged. Note the pulse ox machine.

A crowd of Nepalis under a big tent gave a demonstration. My former wife sat with my daughters among the crowd on folding chairs. I tried to get their attention and they would not show their faces, but I knew it was them. I woke up before it ended, feeling alone and wondering if Dharsha would make it through the night. I thought of what Will had said.

Thursday morning I got to Medical Critical Ward at first light. I expected to see an empty bed. Approaching the room I could see that it was darkened and quiet – I clenched my teeth and steeled myself. *Maybe his brothers had come to get him and take him to the cremation ghat.* But then I could see that Dharsha *was* there with no airway in place. Sleeping quietly on his side. Things were looking up. His brother jumped up when I came in, and told me he had turned the corner overnight. The change in antibiotics was effective, and the night nurses were diligent with the pulmonary care and suctioning. *Thank you God!*

Over the next few days I returned to my routine of clinical supervision on Surgical and only stopped by for a minute or two each day. Dharsha steadily improved though he needed to complete his course of antibiotics. He still could not swallow so the doctors put in a nasogastric tube. In the US, he would have gotten Ensure or some other high calorie formula, but here they gave him watered-down *dal*, greenish lentil soup, that had been pulverized. He resumed swallowing in two more days. Finally, eight days after admission, he was ready for discharge. They sent somebody to bring me to Medical. I arrived to see Dharsha in street clothes. His brother nudged him with an elbow and Dharsha gave me the *namaste* gesture. He still did not know who I was. Seated on the stool next to the bed was a thin woman in a blue and buff-colored *sari*. Her hair was pulled tightly back and she wore red bangles and a *potey* – a green beaded necklace – the color of new rice shoots. She was Dharsha's sister whom I had not met.

I held out my right hand, left hand against my waist, a formal gesture to shake hands. She took my hand in both of hers. We made eye contact as the brother translated for me. She had heard that I had saved Dharsha's life. In a stream of Nepali, she started to thank me. She burst into tears, and burbled the words.

Somebody translated: "You gave us back our brother!"

She wiped her tears on the back of my hand.

She kissed my hand and wept openly.

I did not know what to say. I felt my face getting warm, and I started to blink the tears away. *I knew I would cry if he died, I had not thought I would cry if he lived.* I heard somebody else in the room sniffle.

I thanked Dharsha's sister and stepped outside to compose myself. At the entrance to the ward I allowed myself to weep for a minute. Like Dharsha's sister, I wept tears of actual Joy.

Over the next few days, I was a sort of rock star. People were friendly to me before, but this now took on a new dimension. I never sat by myself anywhere any more, as soon as somebody saw me sit I would be joined and a conversation would start. Walking down the hall, the guys would come up and put their arm on my shoulder so we could walk together in the way the Nepalis do when they are among themselves. The Nepali language tutor wanted to hear the whole story. People would laugh at the slightest funny thing I might say. The hospital Chaplain invited me to his house for dinner. A newcomer to Nepal does not generally receive this kind of personal attention.

This exceeded any fantasy I might have had about working in Nepal, and I loved it. I reflected on the last time I was given this kind of affirmation. *Maybe never.* After Dharsha walked out of the hospital in the company of his family, no matter what else might happen, I had the feeling that it was going to be a great summer.

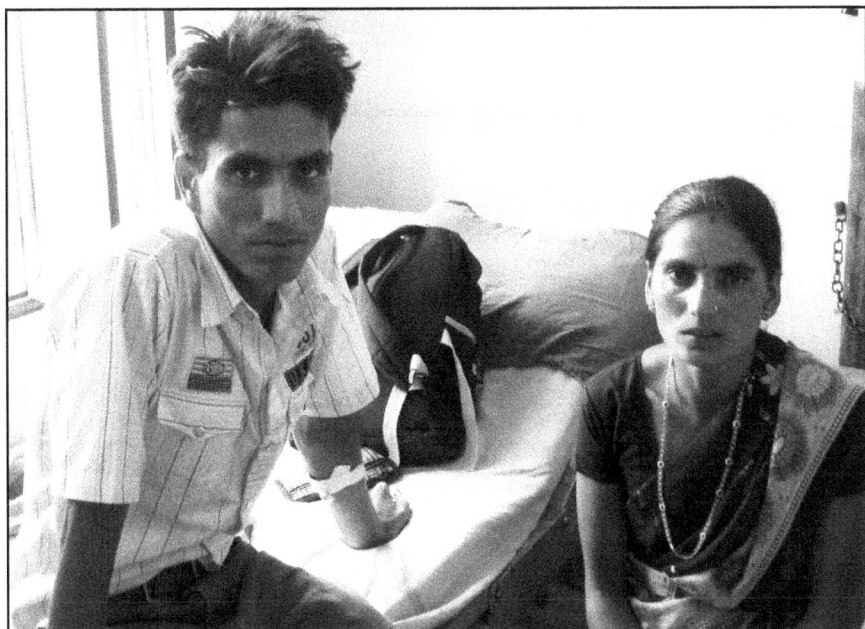

Dharsha and his sister, the day he was discharged.

The Wizard of Auz

For weeks, Samuel had been saying that a really good genito-urinary surgeon would be coming this summer for a few weeks. Samuel prepared for this surgeon's arrival by keeping a list of patients who needed elective genito-urinary surgery. When Dr. Cooper arrived they would be contacted and asked to come to the hospital. Several patients were already at the hospital, waiting.

One such person was a three-year-old boy with chronic urinary tract infections. A few months after birth, he had developed episodes of fever and cloudy urine. They would clear up with antibiotics, but then a new infection would happen soon after the antibiotic was finished. Eventually the urinary tract infection had spread into the child's kidney, a condition known as pyelonephritis. The boy had flank pain and fever. Ultimately, he needed to have a nephrostomy tube put in place, bypassing the bladder altogether. Along the course of his illness, they had done an x-ray with dye to visualize the urinary tract, and it was possible to see that one ureter was normal, about the diameter of a drinking straw, going straight from the kidney to the base of the bladder. The other one was malformed – it looked like it was the size of a garden hose, and took a funny loop. It was attached to the bladder in the wrong location.

Another boy awaiting surgery was born with hypospadias. This is a condition where the urethra exits the penis at the base instead of going all the way to the tip. The child could not pee in the normal way; by that I mean, he could not direct the stream the way all boys do. Later he would not be able to father a child of his own this way.

Also on the list were two children with Hirschsprung's disease. This was a brain-tickler for me, and I needed to look it up, trying to remember the last time I had heard of this problem. It's a disease of the large intestine, and the treatment is to do a "pull through" surgery.

There was a girl who had been born with an anogenital fistula. Her stool exited from a spot inside the vagina, instead of through the anus which seemed too tight. All her life she had experienced frequent urinary tract infections.

In the West, these children would have been referred to a tertiary medical center for treatment. This was not an option here, for the usual reasons. Time, distance, money.

Here is where Dr. Cooper – The Wizard – comes in. I gave him that nickname, but I never used it within his earshot. Weeks before Dr. Cooper arrived, Al and I had been discussing the country we lived in and we decided that Nepal bore more than just a passing resemblance to

Middle Earth. *If this was Middle Earth, then Dr. Cooper, our visiting Aussie surgeon, had to be the Wizard.*

Cooper went to medical school in England and Scotland, and was a professor of Pediatric Surgery at a major center in Australia. He was in his fifties, with a salt-and-pepper beard that reminded me of Henry the Eighth. It's an apt analogy because he also had a courtly air, and a regal demeanor. Not in a condescending way, but there was an aura of confidence, command and generosity about the way he spoke with people. When he turned his face to you and listened, you got the idea that he was giving you his full attention. His face was etched into a permanent wry grin.

This was Cooper's eighth trip to Nepal to do surgery. On previous trips he brought his wife and daughters, but this time his sidekick was a young surgical resident. He would be here for two weeks, present a paper at a medical conference in the UK, and then spend two weeks doing surgery in Gaza on his way home to Oz. "I'm expecting to deal with a bit more politics in Gaza than I get on my trips to Nepal," he said.

He did not jump immediately into surgery. Instead, he spent a part of each day helping the other surgeons and getting to know the Theater team. Then he planned out the careful pre-operative preparation of the children in his care. He ordered more x-rays to get a better view of the ureter and nephrostomy tube on the boy with the recurrent infections. After that, he and Samuel would spend part of the day discussing the ins and outs of the surgeries, so that Samuel could manage the care of the patients afterwards. Cooper knew that the limited resources of the hospital would amplify any miss-steps that might be made and so he was very methodical about his planning. This was a key to his success.

Earlier in the summer the regulars at the Guest House dinner table were the four medical students, myself, and the orthopedic surgeon from Japan. Our Japanese friend would eat quietly but the medical students were louder. Al was animated and we all enjoyed his sense of humor. When Padma came she was the center of attention as the only woman, and she took a lot of good-natured teasing. We would conduct a free-floating discussion, sometimes loudly. Cooper had an aura about him that made the rest of us defer to him to lead the conversation. If there was a lull, we would politely ask him a question to get it started again. There were no side conversations when Cooper was at the table, and it was more formal. Not even Samuel called him by his first name.

One evening after dinner he set up his laptop, and burned some CDs of the digital photos he took that day. Cooper was a photography enthusiast and gave us a tour of the photos he had taken. I was impressed to see his camera, because I knew how expensive it was. There had been one like it on display at the camera store where I bought mine in Honolulu. He also owned a card reader. On the ward I learned that he brought with him a goody bag of specialized equipment such as a pediatric Foley catheters and stents. I asked him how he had obtained these. At first he winked and said they were donated by Theater staff of his home hospital.

I said, "Really?"

Then he laughed and said, "In other words, we nicked 'em!"

When Cooper first arrived, a trauma case came to the ER. A child had been hit by a motorcycle and was brought to Mission Hospital with a serious head injury. The on-call surgeon was one of the Nepalis. When they examined the child they could see that the pupil of one eye was larger than the pupil of the other, and that one arm and leg were weaker than the other. A blood clot on the child's brain was creating pressure – a subdural hematoma. The treatment for this is to relieve the pressure on the brain by cutting a hole in the skull. The Nepali surgeon was hesitant – he had not previously done this procedure. In the meantime the child was dying right before everyone's eyes.

Cooper took the younger surgeon aside and conferred. They took the child quickly to Theater and made an opening in the skull. Cooper would be there to offer advice and aid. They washed out the clot. They also made a small abdominal incision to create a pouch in which to store the cookie-sized piece of bone. It would remain there until it was safe to replace it to the spot from which it originated. The child survived.

Many of Cooper's surgeries were unremarkable because they went so well. Writing the story is like reciting the textbook. Cooper's hypospadias repair was another case. To close the incorrect opening at the base of the boy's penis, Cooper did a circumcision to get some flesh that could be grafted – a sort of a patch over the leak. A day later, I was with one of the students when we removed the dressing. The boy screamed, more in fright than in pain. Once the dressing was off we marveled at the precise small delicate stitches Cooper had placed. The boy's father stood anxiously nearby, and we brought him over to take a look. Cooper told me later that he did this precise work using just the naked eye. "Lots of surgeons use a loupe, a jeweler's lens, but I do not. I suppose I shall use one myself when I get old."

The girl with the ano-genital fistula had a few bumps in her post-operative recovery. When he did the surgery on her anus, Cooper needed to create a double-barreled colostomy, a temporary opening that would divert the patient's stool away from the incision on the ano-genital area while it healed, then ultimately reversed in a few months at which time the patient could resume passing stool the usual way. The surgery went just fine, but the ostomy appliance we were planning to use was too bulky and the girl had thrown it away. That was all we had available, because we had used all of our ostomy appliances for Park's patient. We picked through the trash but it was too late, it had been incinerated. For a couple of days there were no ostomy supplies, and the girl would sit there, holding a towel against her abdomen until it was too soiled, then get another towel. The girl was depressed. We re-assured her that this was temporary. We sent to Kathmandu for more ostomy supplies. There was no medical equipment store in Tansen.

The day came for Cooper to leave. He took the Buck to Kathmandu. Later I heard that he'd enjoyed the UK and made it safely through the time in Gaza as well. He was already planning his ninth trip to Nepal.

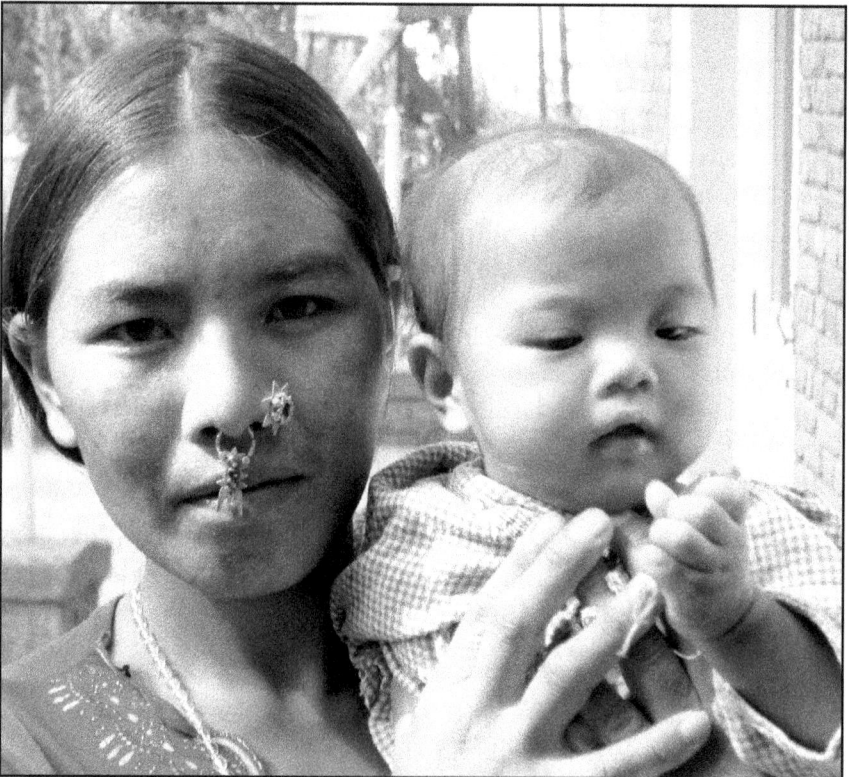

Kusmati and her mother. Note the Magar-style nose jewelry. This is the photo I took on the patio behind the hospital, a few weeks before I started on Pediatrics.

The Mona Lisa of Nepal

At the back of the hospital was a concrete patio with a low wall around it where on the sunny days many patients and relatives would sit to talk or smoke or to just enjoy being outdoors. The patio was on the route between the hospital and the Guest House where I lived, so I would pass by several times a day. Nearby was a nice rhododendron tree I particularly enjoyed, which seemed to be in bloom all summer, a shower of pastel purple blossoms.

One time the construction workers from the ER project took a lunch break on the patio and I watched them do a folk dance. There were twenty workers. Most stood in a circle and sang a song, clapping their hands rhythmically. One man knew all the verses and the rest joined in on a chorus. Men and women took turns in the center, one couple at a time. Not quite touching each other, but very close, giving eye contact and moving their arms to the music. Some of the dance steps involved assuming a low crouch, and they made it look easy as they bounced in this position, but I did not think I could have done that step. The onlookers cheered and laughed, not just the other workers but also the patients outside with their families.

While I was working on the Surgical floor, there was one particular mother and baby who caught my eye as I passed by the patio in the morning. The mother was about thirty- years old. She was a Magar. Most people in Tansen would not have taken a second look at her. At first that was my own reaction. The Magar women dressed as if they were wearing a uniform, though they each managed to convey a sense of personal style. The guidebook described the Magar women as having a "rugged beauty."

She wore a red blouse and red bangles on her wrists, which indicated she was married. Her blouse showed a bit of midriff. It buttoned down the front but she probably never undid the buttons. When she was breastfeeding she would just lift up the bottom hem and allow the baby's mouth to seek out her nipple. Like many Nepali women, breastfeeding did not seem to have any sexual connotations for her. As always, I was careful to avert my eyes when I was a passerby.

For a relatively young woman, she wore unusual jewelry. There were two large nose pieces. Each was made of Newari gold and each was an antique. The septal piece had three rubies on it and hung down from the middle of her nose, overlapping her upper lip. It would have been impossible for her to drink from a cup with that piece in place and I always wondered how she would do it. Drinking straws were not in general use in Nepal. The side piece went through the left nostril. It had one very large ruby. I always wondered how she came by these – probably inherited from her mother. I never saw any other women her age wearing those particular kinds of nose pieces. Only the old women. To eat *dal-bhaat*, women wearing these septal pieces had to bow their heads deeply so that the septal piece would dangle away from the lip.

I learned later that her baby was named Kusmati. Kusmati was cute and had big muscular cheeks like a chipmunk, such as many breastfed infants develop. The baby was about seven-months-old. I could see that the baby had an IV in her wrist and I wondered what was wrong with the child.

Kusmati's mother was Asian of course, as are all Magars. The local *Brahmins* would call her a "*Thapa*." She had long hair, not quite black, but a deep brown, parted in the middle. She seldom smiled but had beautiful teeth. She was of an athletic build, and glided when she walked. She seemed accustomed to carrying a baby on her hip, though she always held this one propped with both arms in front of her, cheek-to-cheek as if to show that she and her daughter were almost Siamese twins.

There was another reason I noticed this particular Magar woman. The look in the eyes, the way she walked, the smile – all these made me think of Celeste, the woman in Honolulu who had given me the Buddhist prayer beads. When I saw Kusmati's mother, I would summon an image of Celeste and think pleasant thoughts.

I wonder how Celeste would like being here in Nepal right now with the rhododendrons and all. Celeste had no children and no boyfriend in sight – but had once told me she wished she had. She could feel her biological clock ticking. "All I am waiting for is the right guy," she would say. This always prompted me to think *what about me?* The Magar woman was built like Celeste, and I could imagine that this baby would be like the one Celeste would be holding if Celeste's wish had come true.

And so when I saw Kusmati's mother I had a feeling of *déjà vu*. It was a pleasant fantasy. She had a musical voice like Celeste, though I don't think I ever said more than a few sentences to her.

One day I saw her at the patio again. I had my camera with me so I stopped and asked, "*Tapaiko photo kijnu sak chu?*" ("Do you mind if I take your picture?"). Kusmati's mother smoothed her hair with one hand then posed proudly with her baby. She nodded her head, *yes*, in the peculiar Nepali way. She still did not smile. She gazed directly into the camera, did not look away or blink. *Like the "Mona Lisa of Nepal."* I took two clear photos and thought these would make a nice thing to show Celeste when I told her the story. My plan was to tell Celeste that she had a double in Tansen, sort of like a science fiction movie plot in which Celeste was a person with a duplicate existence in an alternate universe. Later when

I did show the photos to Celeste she did not see the resemblance, but I still thought it was there.

I was busy on Surgical so I did not give much thought to the Magar woman or her baby for a bit. I assumed that the baby had recovered and been discharged. *Maybe it was pneumonia.*

One day I arrived on the Pediatric Ward and found the Magar woman and her child again. I would always get there early and copy the patient names, room number and diagnoses onto a piece of paper beforehand, because report was in a mixture of Nepali and English. I had learned that if I got off-track with the room number (using the Nepali numbers) I would get hopelessly confused as to which patient was which.

That day, I was still new and the names were not particularly meaningful to me. I knew the usual pattern – we had children with respiratory problems in the first room, communicable diseases in the second room, neonates in the third room, orthopedics in the fourth room, and so on. The nurses tried to cluster the patients this way when they could.

Ward rounds started after report. The day nurses would go from bed to bed to look at each patient. When we entered the room where Kusmati was, I saw Kusmati's mother and I smiled. The mother and baby were sleeping soundly, spooning on the wooden bed. They were in one of the only semi-private rooms in the hospital.

On the Pediatric Ward, there was a specific room in which treatments took place. This was about ten by twelve feet. On one side were a counter, sink and the supplies for dressings. On the other side was a long exam table with a padded surface covered in clear plastic. In Pediatrics there is a rule that the patient's bed is a safe place and that you should never do anything painful there. That way the child can think of their bed as a place to relax. When a procedure is needed, the child is brought to the treatment room. If the child gets a dressing change daily, they get conditioned to cry as soon as they approach the treatment room.

The staff nurse wrote out a list of the day's dressing changes, and I watched her do the first two or three. The next name was Kusmati and there was a lull while the staff nurse prepared the equipment tray and covered it with a sterile drape. She did not have such good English and my Nepali was terrible so this was done with minimal conversation. Then she went out to get Kusmati's mother. It was the Magar woman, and at first I smiled when she came in the room. *Here was the woman who reminded me of Celeste... And her baby.* Thinking of Celeste made me smile.

Kusmati's mother sat down on the stool next to the treatment table and adjusted the waterproof sheet on her lap, then held Kusmati there.

The staff nurse lifted the baby's hospital gown, exposing gauze dressings on both legs. There were large spots where blood and some kind of thick, yellowish fluid were soaking through. The bandages did not extend all the way to her feet, and I was jolted to realize that *this baby had no toes.* None. Her feet were two stumps. The skin on the soles of her feet was parchment-paper thin and crusty like old sunburn. This part at least, had already been grafted to form a covering of skin. Kusmati squirmed and I could see the tarsal bones on the top of both her feet working like worms in a bag. She was squirming in pain as the nurse matter-of-factly poured saline on the leg dressings to loosen them from the burn wounds and graft sites that covered both legs and buttocks.

I looked at the missing toes. I looked at the squirming feet, writhing in pain. She was kicking. At first I looked at the dressings coming off – gauze covering a raw surface about the size of a dessert plate on her shin, another on the thigh, and two more of equal size on the other leg. The dressing stuck and the nurse dripped more saline. The saline became tinged with the blood and pus, running down the waterproof sheet onto the floor. The baby had a distinctive high-pitched cry and she was crying now. I averted my eyes – and looked directly into the gaze of Kusmati's mother, who was watching me while she cooed to her baby and tried to distract the baby by offering her breast to the baby's screaming mouth. Milk was dripping. The baby clutched the breast tightly with both hands and worked it roughly like it was play dough. The same solemn expression. *I now knew what it was. It was not an expression of serenity. Not a Mona Lisa.* It was a face of sorrow as she held her baby every day, mixed with determination as she let down milk while the baby cried. *What if that was Celeste?*

I held her gaze for about a second but it seemed like an hour. Then she wiped away a tear. I could feel warmth in my chest as if I had just jumped from a sauna into an ice cold lake. I mopped my forehead with my bandana, got up and left the room. I walked down the hall and down the stairs to the patio in back. I took deep breaths. *O God, how could this happen? God! How could you let this happen? God! How could a child suffer this way?* The tears started but they would not flow. I stood there clenching my fists. I keep my fingernails short as all good nurses do, but if they had been long I am sure I would have pierced both my palms with them. I asked myself what I had just seen, and had a talk with "Little Joe."

And then after a few minutes on the patio I went back. By this time the nurse had moved on to the next child. This case happened to be a tubercular leg wound in an eight-year-old in which about six inches of shinbone was exposed. No problem. This kid was brave and did not cry. He was with his grandfather, not his mom.

It was clear that we were going to do Kusmati's dressing every day for the next few weeks but for this day we had finished the list of dressings.

Later, I sat at the desk in my apartment at the Guest House, sunlight on the page of my open journal as I wrote. Music wafted through the window. One of the Nepali interns was playing the radio; it was an American pop tune. I froze for a second, listening intently. *Back Street Boys*. It was *"Tell Me Why –"*

(Tell me why?)
Ain't nothing but a heartache
(Tell me why?)
Ain't nothing but a big mistake
(Tell me why?)
I never want to hear you say
I want it that way.

Like a lot of American pop tunes that made it to Nepal, it was eight-years old. This song was about a failed relationship and lost love. I had this thought right then that like many love songs, it could express my thoughts about my relationship with God at that moment. *You could make it a prayer. A prayer that asks tell me why? Tell me why God would abandon somebody.* To this day, when I hear that song I find that I recall the time and place when it took on this new meaning for me. And, the feelings return. And, I need to talk with Little Joe... and tell him its okay.

Over the next month, I was to change Kusmati's dressing many times with the nursing students, and look into the eyes of her mother, and each time think again of my friend Celeste and the time she told me she wanted children. We started to routinely give Kusmati a drug named ketamine before each dressing change so that her pain would be lessened, which helped everyone to get through it a little better.

For me, I had been enjoying a wave of popularity since the outcome of the snakebite incident, but the day I saw Kusmati's legs the first time, was the precise moment that the positive vibe came clattering to a halt.

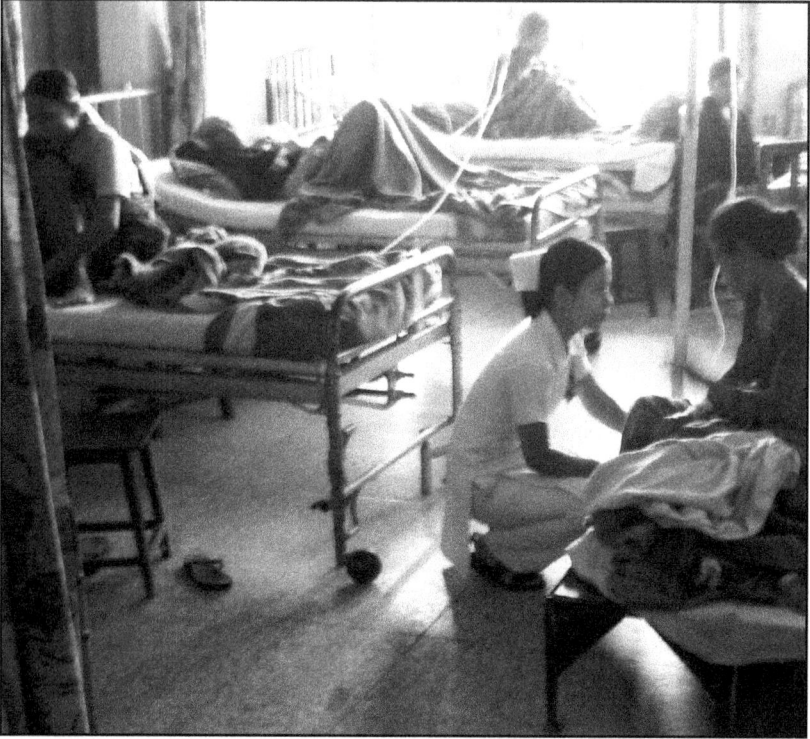

One of the rooms on Medical, kneeling student is speaking with a patient who spent the night on a pallet.

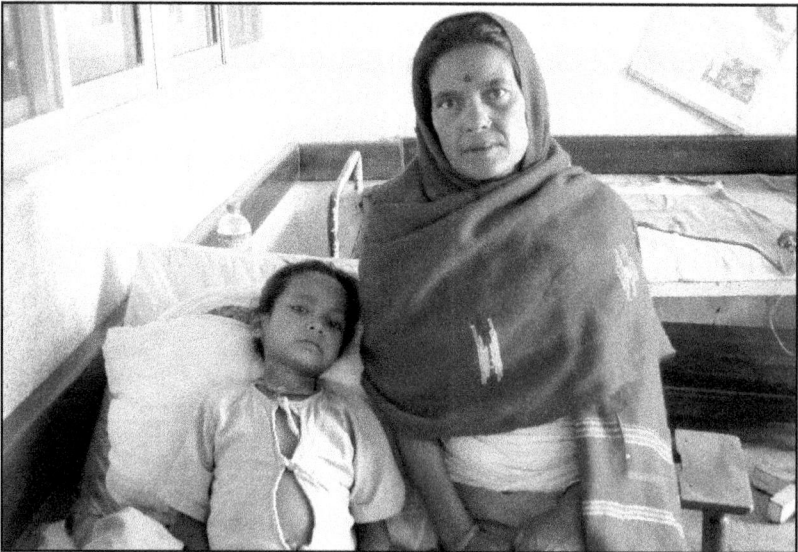

This child was admitted with severe infestation of intestinal worms. The mother wears a Magar outfit with shawl and Patuka though the temperature is about eighty degrees fahrenheit.

Children on Pallets

Pediatric and Surgical were in two different buildings connected by a short corridor like the letter "H". In the middle of the corridor was the double door to the ramp that led to Orthopedics and Medical, one floor below Pediatrics. In summer this door was always open. At the busiest part of the summer, there were eight pediatric patients on pallets in addition to the fifty in beds. This day the pallets made a line like dominoes or boxcars, starting in Pediatrics, past the door, almost to the Surgical floor. One of the long term missionaries said this was the most she had ever seen.

This was the busiest corridor in the hospital, with a continual stream of foot traffic. The children on pallets tended to be ortho patients with fresh fractures or freshly reduced fractures. They were in pain. One or both parents would be sitting there with them. The only way to get to the nursing station was to walk past the people sitting on the pallets. The crowd conveyed an idea of the huddled masses of humanity. "The Bus Station Effect" once again.

The nursing school did not teach Pediatrics year-round. Tansen Nursing School used the curriculum from CVEVT, the Nepal educational agency that dictated a standard course plan. Pediatrics was placed in the second year of the nursing program, and it was taught for four months. Here it seemed that pre-monsoon was probably the busiest season for Pediatrics. Each nursing student did a one-month rotation, and there were four groups of students. The age of the students was seventeen. They appeared on the Clinical floor on day one, before any of the class room lectures had begun.

A child is never given the adult dose of any medication, and every nurse must know how to double check the doctor's calculation as to a safe proportionate medication dose. In a well organized nursing school, when a student first performs this, she is watched very closely and given one-to-one supervision. At Mission Hospital, this meant that when one student in the group was giving medications, the other nine would largely be working with the staff nurses thus not getting the attention of the pediatric nursing instructor. Two faculty were needed.

In June on Surgical I was covering faculty vacations. First one then the other. But by the end of June all the vacations were over. Surgical would be fully staffed. They had to decide how best to use me. In mid-June, around the time of the snakebite incident, the Principal and a couple of the older faculty of the School of Nursing got together at a meeting to discuss what to do with me.

One of the two regular faculty members on Pediatrics had just gotten married and moved to Kathmandu. Now, there was only Sanjita, the youngest faculty member. A big chunk of Sanjita's time each day was devoted to medication preparation and administration supervision. If I joined her there, we could do more procedures with the students. Besides, I got along well with Norma and Samuel, the two pediatricians. Pediatrics was busy.

One of the senior faculty members told me about the personnel meeting the next day. At first I was surprised that I was not invited, but then maybe that was how it worked in Nepal. I knew very well that the leaders of the hospital and the nursing school were not shy about re-assigning people if it was warranted. I saw this process firsthand with Park. He was re-assigned with lightning speed. *This was as it should be. Just because a person was a volunteer and a foreigner would not guarantee that they would be put in any kind of responsible position.* In that respect, getting assigned to Pediatrics was an acknowledgement of my skills. I was being jumped ahead of another foreign faculty, an actual missionary, who had been at the Nursing School a year, for instance, and wanted to be on Pediatrics. She was very unhappy and complained bitterly. But the Principal of the school told her that she needed more experience. Maybe next year.

Then I needed to think about teaching Pediatrics again. Much of nursing depends on the language skill of the nurse, and this is even more important in Pediatrics. To be honest I was a bit afraid of making a mistake or overlooking some symptom of a pediatric disease. During my brief orientation in early June, I saw how busy it could be on Pediatrics. To be present during the death of a child is particularly disturbing. I was wondering if I was ready for more emotionally turbulent events. I am more comfortable taking care of adults.

On the other hand I also felt a sense of duty to go where they asked me to go. Sanjita was young. She was a Tansen Nursing School grad, "Batch of 2005." *Another quaint expression they used.* She graduated at the top of her nursing class and was very intelligent. For example, she knew what *montegia* was. She and I could make a great team. I realized that for the first time in my life I would be taking direction from a person the same age as my younger daughter – twenty-two. Sanjita was descended from the settlers in the Terai who had emigrated from India. Sanjita was Indian in racial origin, not Aryan like the *Brahmins* and *Chhetris*.

It would not have surprised me to see Sanjita's photo in Nepal tourism magazines, that's how attractive she was – raven hair, big brown doe-eyes, mocha complexion and a way of smiling at you innocently when you talked with her, eyes scanning nervously. She had perfect teeth and smiled often. Sanjita wore her hair in a severe bun at the nape of the neck, like all the other nurses. She told me that in her city in the *Terai*, the lowland near the border with India, the women all wore their bun at the top of the head; but that people here would laugh at her if she wore it that way. She did not wear a *tika*, and I wondered whether she was Christian or Hindu. Later I asked her and she said she had tried Christianity until recently, but now that her Christian friend was married and moved away, she decided to return to the Hindus. Unlike most Hindu nurses, she did not wear a nose piercing, just a faint scar on the left nares where it had been. "I don't wear much jewelry."

At first, Sanjita called me by the same name the students did, "Joe Sar." "Sar" was the way they pronounced "sir." I started calling her "Sanjita Ma'am" in reply, mimicking the formal honorific tone used by the students when they addressed us. She blushed. Sanjita was soft spoken with me but not afraid to take charge of the students. She knew the routine of the ward very well since she had trained there not too long ago. She was usually just a tad late for report every day. One day I noticed a small oily stain on the back apron of her uniform. It was there each of the next two days. It was evidence that she did not wash her uniform or change it every day. I don't think that was unusual. Maybe she only owned one uniform.

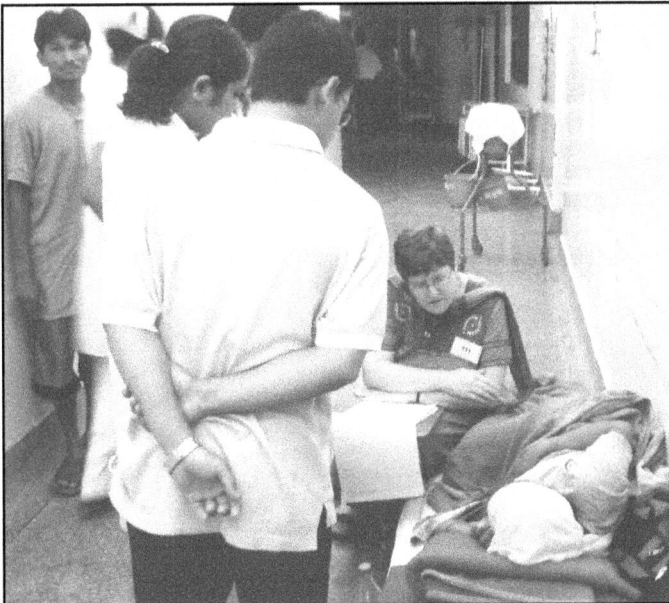

Attending physician making morning rounds with patient on pallet. Note hand washing station in back.

The Students Buckle Down

There is an outdoor patio near the corridor that connects the Pediatric Ward and Surgical. Most days, the railing is hung with newly washed red *saris* and other clothes items drying in the sun. It was usually unoccupied when I came in for the day. This day I knew that people were there, as soon as I passed the rhododendron tree, and the sense of dread grew as I came up the ramp from the Guest House. *What is that godawful wailing?* I stopped. The patients on the pallets in the corridor were quiet, looking back as I surveyed the scene. *The patio.* On the patio was a group of women, about a dozen, so close together they might have been a rugby scrum. In the center was a woman about my age who was removing the bangles from her wrists, throwing them down, and stomping them. She was too weak to stand, and her friends were supporting her – literally and figuratively. I kept walking toward Pediatrics. The night nurse told me a patient died in the ER. The chorus of wailing continued for a half hour.

Shortly thereafter I met the ten students in our Pediatric group. These were the second-year "batch." They were all seventeen-years old. This group had been on Surgical and Medical the previous year, doing the dressings and medications. With a year under their belt they were more confident.

The first day with the students, the corridor was still clogged with all the overflow pallets in the corridor. One mother was from the Terai. Sanjita knew I was watching her as she knelt to speak with the woman in Hindi. Later, Sanjita smiled as she told me "I speak four languages – English, Nepali, Hindi, and the language of my caste." She learned Hindi because she watched a lot of Bollywood MTV. The census that day was fifty-eight patients on Pediatrics. Sanjita and I divided the workload so that each day starting about nine, I would supervise dressing changes. The ward staff gave us a list of dressings that needed to be done, and the students divided them up. There were about ten dressings to do. I already knew what some of the dressings would be like, after observing the staff when I spent a day there the previous week. Watching the first burn dressing change, on the child with the burned legs, had been a shock to me.

Over the next few hours we dealt with one crying and struggling child after another. The students did not know how to approach the children in a way that would minimize the terror of anticipating a dressing change. They did not know how to instruct the mother to position a child so that it would be still. We had one scalp dressing where the Theater staff had applied the old-fashioned extra-sticky cloth tape to the scalp without properly cutting the hair first, so we had to cut the hair of the child to get the tape off. The mom would not hold the child's head still and the child wagged back and forth. I think we nicked the scalp a half dozen times. Each time I clenched my teeth.

The students thought they did not really need to move to the treatment room for certain dressings. Sometimes, such as when the child was in traction, moving to the treatment room was not feasible. One of the students assured me that she could do a particular dressing change on a child in the ward, even though I politely suggested that we move to the treatment room. She acted confident as she told me it was okay, and I acquiesced. There were no privacy drapes on the ward and there were ten other patients.

The child's cries summoned the typical audience that gathers whenever anything interesting happens in Nepal. As the child alternately screamed and whimpered, about fifteen parents and passersby gathered around us. Both the student and I broke out into a sweat as we fumbled through the dressing procedure while the audience watched. They seemed to be commenting on us like spectators at a cricket match. Later, I took that student aside and told her in no uncertain terms that tomorrow we would do the dressing in the treatment room, period. I did not want her to question me ever again. From then on I was more assertive with that student.

The age of the child dictates the approach to use when doing a procedure. It was clear that the students had not developed any strategies to minimize pain and terror - they had not even thought of this. I asked them if they had ever heard the term "Stranger Anxiety" and they had not. So I assigned them to look it up. On the Surgical Ward where they had been, the patients were adults. The Nepali adults on Surgical were resigned to the idea that they would not be getting much pain medicine. The students had not really dealt with the issue of pain and terror in children even though they had done many dressings on adults.

We got through the list by one in the afternoon, and I left to have my language lesson. My mind was churning and I needed to go for a walk to just think about something else for a bit. That night I lay awake and perseverated on all the crying and struggling during the day. The crying had reverberated throughout the ward all day long, and I was replaying the events. In the end, I was harsh on myself as to why it was unsatisfactory. The obvious answer was that I should have planned better and done more to take charge, not to let the students lead it until they had more experience. There was nobody to blame but myself. The students did not know any better. If they were to learn, I had to teach them. I had gotten into Pediatrics without any preconceived notions as to what it would be like, but now that I had been with the students for a day, I needed to get actively engaged in leading the students.

The next morning the students started out smiling when they saw me, then I took the group aside and laid down some ground rules for the dressings. I held up their textbook and told them they needed to start studying it. Use the treatment room, close the door and control the access. Premedicate. Teach the mom how to hold the baby. Restrain if needed. Think about when to explain. Use distraction techniques. I said all this with a grim expression on my face. By the time I was through, the students were very serious. The fun was over. Pediatrics was not going to be as easy as they may have thought. They were going to see a different side of me than their friends on Surgical had seen.

It was still a struggle, and that day was only a bit better than the previous day. For me, it was draining. Each student might do only one or two dressings a day, but I was with all of the dressing changes, ten or more a day. This took about five hours a day. *Who needs this!*

When people choose their life work, they all have a vision or fantasy about what they will be doing when they are at work. It's a way to write the script of your life, which validates your self-image and helps you keep going. We all have these scripts whether we know it or not. I had a pretty straightforward idea of who I was and why I was working in health care. For me, the daydream that sustained me was one in which I was a person who worked hard to protect and rescue helpless people. Other persons may choose a different day dream by which to guide their life – maybe being wealthy or powerful – but this heroic rescue fantasy was my personal favorite.

And now I was leading a team of seventeen-year-old girls, doing one daily wound dressing after another, on a busy Pediatric Ward. It was a big challenge to this daydream. *Nobody chooses this. Nobody in their right mind decides to dedicate their life to intentionally inflict suffering on children all day.* The circumstances made me feel sort of trapped, like I was stuck doing this. A few times I started to talk with Sanjita or with Rati, who coordinated the second-year courses. Each time they were very complimentary about how well I was doing. They pointed out that in all fairness, the lecture component of the course started the same week as the first day, and so it was true that early on the students did not know the theory to back up why we did things a certain way, but they would catch up quickly. Rati was a beautiful woman and she knew it.

She smiled and fluttered her eyelashes at me as she spoke. "It is an honor to for the Tansen Nursing School faculty to work with you, Joe." and "You are helping the team so much. The first year students and third year students have learned so much from you on Surgical, now you can also work with the second-year batch here on Pediatrics." *She knew exactly how to butter me up.*

At dinner that evening, Al played "I'm Thinking of a Person" with the children of a visiting UMN person who was in town for a few days. Padma blushed while she gave us an announcement. That day she delivered her first baby, a girl. It was a first-time mother, a *primipara* in obstetrical parlance. The first baby from any given mother is not as easy to predict as a second or third delivery would have been. The labor progressed normally, and Ellie had been in the background, consulting when asked. Padma managed the mother through transition and pushing, which would be a milestone in the education of any young doctor, and assessed the newborn after delivery. The patient was in active labor for about five hours, and there were a few twists and turns along the way, which she shared in detail as if she herself had given birth. She made good decisions along the way and it sounded like she did a good job directing the team.

Padma was radiant with pride. We all congratulated her. Al and I teased her about whether the baby would be named after her. Regretfully, no. But since the new baby girl would not get a name until she was eleven days old, the door of possibility was still open.

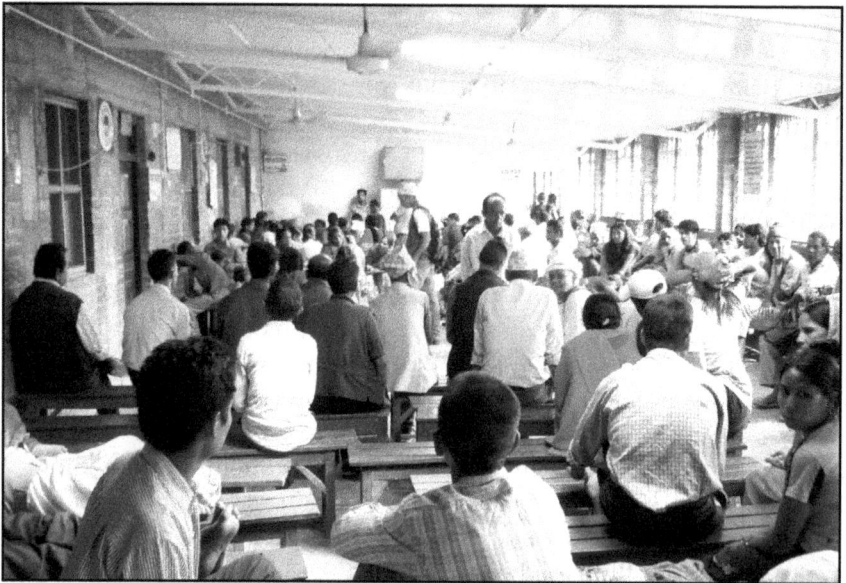

Photo facing page: The waiting room outside the ER and clinic. Due to the endemic TB in the region, I always figured that there was at least one active case among the people sitting there on any given day.

An Unexpected Person Outside the ER

I knew that I was not smiling as much or joking with the students the way I had when I was on Surgical. But it is not as if I was new to health care or to death. I started doing ICU nursing in 1978, but I was never involved in pediatric burn care before. There seemed to be a lot of burn injuries. When I asked why, people told me that it was because of the lack of electricity in the rural areas. At night, people burn kerosene in makeshift lamps to light up the house. It gets dark around seven o'clock in this part of the tropics, year round.

Mister Spirituality. My former wife used that nickname for me. She seemed to dismiss my attempts to be introspective about faith, and at the time I did not have the words to describe what I needed to do to find peace. She would use this nickname every now and then, sarcastically. I ignored it at the time but there was a cumulative effect of shutting off the things we could share. Anger and sarcasm will close doors that a couple might need to leave open in times of difficulty. *I was surely on a faith journey now.*

Here in Nepal I wished that I could go back in time to a place before I started to question God's plan for people on earth. *Not possible.* I wished I could go back to a time when my wife and lover could be a confidante and supporter on spiritual issues. *Hell, I would have settled if she supported me on any issues.* I was trying to call up my Buddhist teachings. *The past is gone. Get anger out of your life.* It occurred to me that I needed a good old fashioned hug from somebody. *I was not going to get one here.*

The day after I saw the leg burns of Kusmati, we were dealing with a newborn baby that was dying of tetanus. This is rarely seen in the US anymore, but in this case the umbilical cord was severed with a piece of sharpened bamboo. The neonate was born at home and was now eleven days old. He was vigorous at first, and then developed a sort of a hunched neck like he was having a permanent cramp there. He was febrile and not able to suck, so he was being fed through a tube. He was having muscle spasms and seizures, and seemed to be trembling all the time.

At first the baby was getting intravenous valium but this was not working to control the seizures so Doctor Norma was going to switch to intravenous magnesium. She spent some time with the interns going over the dose for intravenous magnesium in an infant, because the literature was unclear as to this indication. It occurred to me that it was obscene for us to be having this kind of discussion; this baby should not be dying of this illness. His seizures became longer and more frequent, and he died before the time of the second dose so it was a moot point. We did not resuscitate him.

After work I planned to go to the *Bajar* to collect the first of the *cholos* I had ordered from Kusiram. It would be a pleasant twenty-minute walk as usual. There were limited ways to exit the hospital compound. The lower gate was partly blocked by the construction project. Most people would go through the upper gate and past the ER entrance. Each of these gates was guarded by a *Chowkidar* in khaki uniform and black *topi*. In mid-afternoon there was always a crowd outside the upper entrance. Today there were about fifty people milling around. Many employees rode motorcycles to work, and about ten were parked off to the side right next to the door, like horses in a corral. There were also about ten cars parked willy-nilly near the gate, a few with doors hanging open though their drivers were off somewhere, some homeless people that had been sleeping by the door lately were awake and squatted there looking forlorn, and people smoking there because they were not allowed to smoke in the waiting room. I needed to push through the crowd to make my way.

As I pushed, I bumped against a hospital stretcher. There was somebody laying on it, but the side rails were not in the up position. And the person was in a shroud. Dead. *There in plain view, was a shrouded body on a stretcher.* It was unmistakable. White sheets with red twine around the neck, across the chest and around the knees. With all the people present, there did not seem to be any particular person who was attending this particular dead body. *What the heck?!* I stopped for a moment, looked around, and kept walking. I supposed it was waiting to be picked up.

I wanted to take my mind off the heavy subjects, but the sight of this shrouded body made me think. *One more. Where did this one come from? And I do not even have a clue as to who this one was.* As I walked, I thought back to the idea of a Good Death. In the US, a dying person could sign up for hospice services, which would allow them to die in comfortable surroundings. With a planned death, you got your affairs in order, your pain was controlled, and the family would gather around while you took your last breaths, waving goodbye as you faded away. In the hospice movement, a Good Death was the goal, even though it might not happen as often as the philosophers would wish.

In Nepal – never. More often death was ugly. The patient would be younger than expected. The nurses and doctors would be doing things to try to prevent the person's heart from stopping while the relatives worked on their unresolved issues, and eventually the team would confront the biological fact that the machine we call a body would no longer function, for whatever reason. As I passed people on the way to the *Bajar*, I found myself looking at them and predicting how they would each die. This one? Looking thin – maybe TB. That one? Lung disease. This one? Maybe contaminated drinking water or a car accident. That baby? Typhoid. There were so many ways to die in Nepal, and only a few countries with worse statistics. *Tell me why......* I meditated on the tune as I walked.

When I got to the *Bajar* I paid Kusiram for the *cholo*. Then I also bought the petticoats for my Magar outfits at another place, after that some Cadbury's chocolate, stopping to eat some right there in the street. Regular American chocolate would melt at the usual temperature of Nepal in pre-monsoon. Cadbury's seemed to have a different composition that made it less gooey in the tropics. I brought the *cholo* back to the Guest House, but I was worried about the size. After all, I had only given Kusiram the approximate size; he did his best to accommodate me but he did not know how to translate an American size eight into the usual Nepali measurements. Most of the time the person for whom he was making the clothes would be standing right there, but not this time.

At dinner, we discussed the body outside the ER. We all saw him laying there. Al told us the body was that of a forty-year-old man who died on Medical of a brain hemorrhage. The relatives brought the body to the door then left it there while they went to make a bamboo litter. Normally bodies would go out the lower gate but this was not possible due to the construction project. The relatives returned later, put the body straight on the litter, then led a small procession north to Bagnas, the closest spot for cremation. I was surprised at this, because it was a hike of about three miles on a hot day. I wondered how long it took and whether they had enough people to take turns. Nepalis are champion walkers.

For some reason the conversation soon changed to movies, and Al was conducting a toot on the idea of what exactly constituted a "chick flick." We discussed the elements of emotion and intrigue that made chick flicks a distinct genre. Padma was of course, the final judge. The medical students referred to movies whose names I did not recognize, which made me feel a bit old.

I had this bright idea that I would ask Padma to model the *cholo* for me – she was about the same size as my older daughter. She was shy about it at first but tried it on while the guys all watched. It showed her bosom off very well, but the arms were slightly short and the shoulders were small, and so I decided to go back and ask Kusiram to make some larger ones. In the meantime, Padma still looked nice in it and seemed to preen as she wore it, smoothing the stomach and standing a little more upright. We looked at her. We were all reminded that she was not quite one of the guys. She looked back at us looking at her in that light and she blushed. I made a mental note to order a *cholo* for her as well.

Advice From an Aussie

Near the Orthopedic Ward there was a six-bed room set aside for adult burn victims. We usually had about five patients there, in various stages of skin grafting. The adult Burn Unit was equipped with special shower stalls where the patients could sit while they used tweezers to pick the dead skin from their own wounds, and each was given pain medication before their daily session. Tansen Nursing School assigned a faculty member to work with students there – a nurse from Oz, Barbara. She was Ellie's wife. Barbara went to nursing school in Sydney. Here she worked part-time since she was home schooling their three children. She was tall, blonde and vivacious with full lips and a ready smile. Her Oz accent was like Ellie's and it often took a minute for me to understand her. When she spoke it caused me to stop and re-translate her words in to my own regional (American) dialect of English. Her expression included the eyebrow-raised look that made one think she was always surprised. *How do the Aussies all seem to work their facial muscles in that fashion?* She was a fan of cricket – I never knew what The Ashes were until she told me one time. Barbara had a positive outlook on life. She did not appear to be troubled by her involvement in burn care.

I told her what I was thinking and that I was depressed. She told me to pray more. *Fair enough.* Her suggestion gave me a mixture of responses all at once, which I glossed over. I said nothing because I did not want to offend her. She cocked her head and seemed to take a careful look at me, as if to read any subtle signs I might be giving off. The gesture reminded me of a parrot that was checking out a person who had come too near the cage. She then asked how long I had been in town and how many days I had worked.

"There's your problem Joe. You haven't even been out of Tansen since you arrived. Too many six-day work weeks. Sounds as though you need a trip to Pokhara. A boat ride on the *Phewa Taal* and a few beers in a proper pub would do you some good. "

"Barbara, I thought you were a missionary – what would the kids say if they heard you tell me to have a beer?"

"Joe, I told you to pray first, didn't I? Australia could never have been civilized without beer."

Despite my initial reaction to the prayer idea, I did mull it over. I would need to go to Pokhara sometime in July to renew my visa anyway – I had a sixty day visa but was staying for eighty-four days. Maybe I should go to Pokhara sooner as opposed to later. Pokhara was a seven-hour bus ride away from Tansen. I had not ridden on the public bus system yet. The medical students from the Guest House were in Pokhara that very week – I would get some tips from them when they returned. Barbara told me there was a hotel in Pokhara that catered to Christian Missionaries by giving steep discounts.

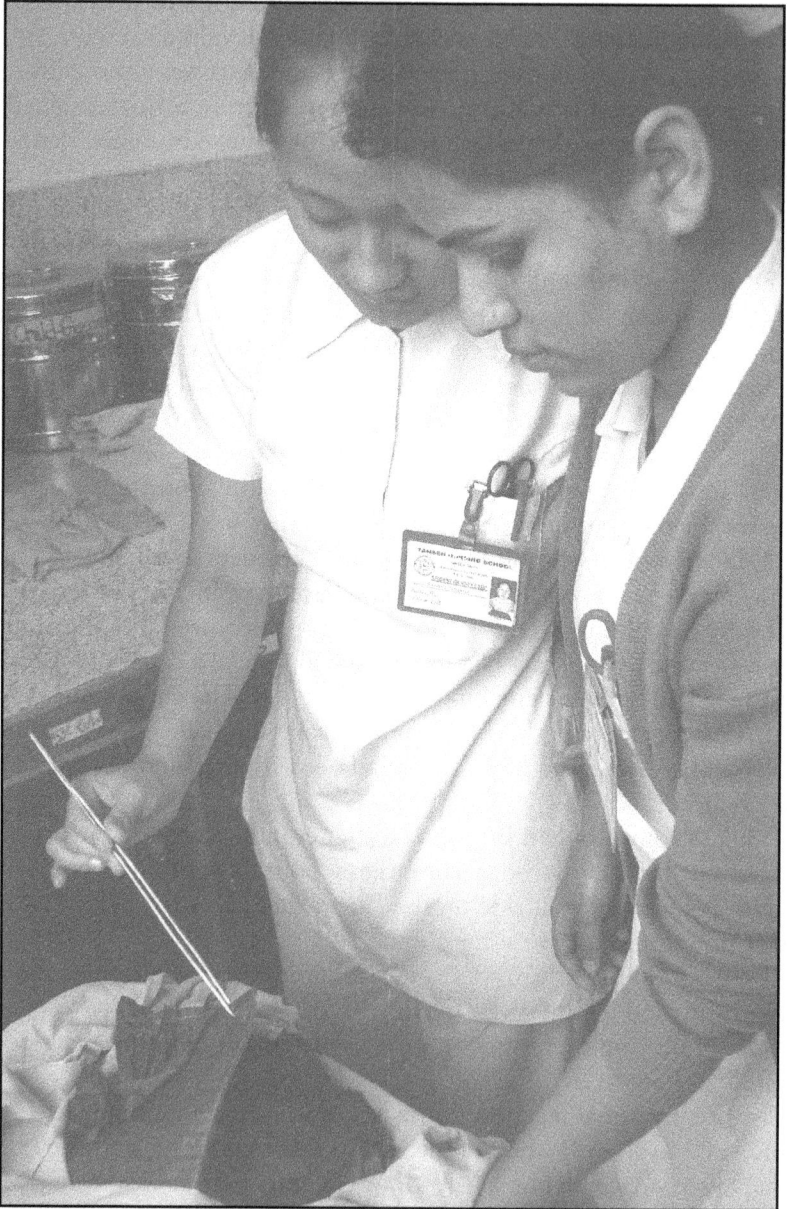

Two nursing students on Pediatrics, picking through some banana leaves that have been sterilized for future use on a burn victim.

New Uses for Banana Leaves

During the days when I was engulfed in the care of Dharsha, the snakebite victim, Mission Hospital hosted a visitor who was an expert in burn care. Pokhara is a much bigger town than Tansen, and Pokhara also has its own hospital with a Burn Unit. The doctor in charge of the Burn Unit there arrived in Tansen to do a toot on wound care. She came for three days and stayed at the Guest House with her family. When she came, Mission Hospital reviewed its practices on burn care. The most important change would be the use of banana leaves. Pokhara used banana leaves in their burn treatment protocol and it was working well for them.

I wondered whether a botanist used a special name for the anatomical part of the plant that we were calling a leaf. *Would it be more accurate to call it a "frond?"* They are large, maybe a foot across and five or six feet long. While still on the plant, they are shiny and sort of waxy. The waxiness makes them waterproof, and the size allows you to cut them into various shapes. We could see a dozen banana plants right outside the window of Pediatrics.

A burn wound is warm and moist, and provides ideal conditions in which to grow bacteria. Normally, a special cream with silver nitrate is used to kill bacterial growth. The silvadene cream is slathered on and covered with squares of gauze, then wrapped with rolls of gauze. The gauze can stick to the wound so tightly that it rips the surface when it is removed, causing pain like a blowtorch. To loosen it, a mild saline solution is poured onto the outer gauze. The saline will loosen the places where the gauze has stuck to the burn wound surface.

The problem with this way of doing it, as explained by the doctor from Pokhara, is that the outer gauze often becomes wet – perhaps with the patient's urine or feces. Gauze does not serve as a moisture barrier. At each dressing change you remove bacteria but also more bacteria are introduced into the wound. The wound starts to smell. The patient is in danger of developing infection, sepsis and eventually death.

If the victim appeared in the ER with burns covering more than forty percent of their body, they would not be admitted to the hospital – they would be sent home to die there instead. This policy comes across as heartless and cruel, but it was based on the harsh reality of survival and resource expenditure. Skin grafts are harvested from areas of intact skin using a surgical implement that resembles a fancy cheese slicer. Any given victim needs an area of intact skin from which to obtain donor grafts that would be moved to cover the burned area. If the area of intact skin does not exceed the area of burned skin, there is not enough tissue available. In early June when I oriented to the ER, I once watched the staff carefully calculate the exact percentage of burn involvement when a pediatric burn victim arrived. The child was admitted, but for a moment it looked as though she exceeded the percentage. The ER staff double checked their assessment.

The new way to do burn dressings would be to put on the silvadene, then cover the wound with a banana leaf, then wrap the gauze to hold the banana leaf in place. The banana leaf did not stick and served as a moisture barrier. I suppose in the West they use saran wrap for this purpose. I had not anticipated the need to be well informed on current burn care before going to Nepal, and I wished I knew what they really used in the West. Saran Wrap would be ideal. I was sure that there was some kind of sterile version.

At Mission Hospital, there was an official job category called the *peon*. This was a group of men who wore powder-blue uniforms. The peons did various lifting jobs, such as sending a three-man crew to replace the oxygen tanks when they were empty. They would show up to lift the patients, especially when the patient was of low caste.

Here was a job for the *peons*. We sent one of the peons out with a ladder to a nearby banana plant. He harvested an armful of leaves for us. The charge nurse inspected each leaf. The leaves were sent to Theater to be sterilized. They came back wrapped in blue cloth, and when we opened the cloth, I was reminded of huge cigar tobacco leaves. The leaves had lost their sheen but were still water proof.

We started to use this treatment on Kusmati, the baby with no toes. We also used it on another infant girl on Pediatrics whose third-degree burns covered the backs of her thighs and extended on to her buttocks near the anus. On this child, the pattern of burn injury was a clear indication that the child must have been in a sitting position when she was burned. It was as if there had been a puddle of kerosene just before the flash, everything below the waterline was affected. Every time this other baby moved her bowels, the wound and the dressing got contaminated. In both cases, using the leaves instead of the gauze seemed a lot less painful. The census remained high. We waited for the monsoon to come. Looking south, we could see billowing clouds over the ridge in the direction of Butwal, in the Terai. There, the temperature was one-hundred-fourteen degrees. A fine red dust covered everything and the housekeeping staff spent part of each day squatting with a wet rag to dampen the floor and collect the dust. If you weren't careful you might trip over them.

Fourth of July

Fourth of July fell on a Wednesday in 2007, but there were too many work conflicts among the Americans in Tansen, so it was agreed that we would hold the proper festivities on the sixth of July. After all, the International Date Line was involved somehow, though we could never quite figure out exactly how. Plus we were so far from the "good ol' USA" that if we all agreed not to tell anybody, the people back home would never have any reason to suspect that we skipped the actual holiday. Almost all of the med students had gone to Pokhara, so there were only eight American adults. We invited the Canadians and the Aussies to join us, former colonists in their own right. Turns out that the Brits in Tansen also enjoyed a good party and there were no hard feelings, so they also came. And how could we forget our staunch allies, the South Koreans? In the end, every *videshi* who was not on call was there.

The party was to be held in the Gairegau complex about a mile from the hospital. This was a collection of adjacent houses where many of the senior doctors with families lived. These houses were built in the 1920s and were classics of neo-colonial design, built with brick and fronted with Georgian columns. Each house featured a wide front porch, and a perennial garden along the side. There was a nice square grassy yard in between the houses. It would have been ideal for croquet, but nobody had a croquet set in Tansen. I told Will I was going to bring my trumpet, but he cautioned me not to play until after the meal. "It's sure to call out the neighborhood kids and we can't feed everyone who comes."

I got there after spending the day in Clinical, while the women were still setting the food on the table. I caught my breath, inhaled sharply. Above the table, hanging limp in the still air was an American flag. *Old Glory in a faraway land.* It was a good-sized flag, three by five feet. Tears came to my eyes. I had heard that people abroad have this reaction but had not considered it for myself. I felt like saying the Pledge of Allegiance, as if I was back in sixth grade. I thought of happy Fourth of July celebrations in Skowhegan, Maine when my kids were little and my family was not spread all over the map. The group gathered around to make social conversation while the food was being prepared.

While we were having soft drinks, Will came up to me and we made small talk. He asked, "Do you have a job in the states?" *Odd question, I thought he knew at least that much about me.*

"Yes, I am only here for the summer, I am going back to my teaching job in mid-August." He seemed a bit surprised. We worked alongside each other during the whole episode with Dharsha. Every time I talked with Will it had been about the medical care, strictly business. I did not take the time to get to know him the way I had with Samuel. So I told him a bit about my job, my family, and my life in Hawaii. He did not know I was divorced.

Samuel was late, but arrived in time to get a plate while there was still food on the table. He took me aside to tell me that, by the way, on Pediatrics there was a child with meningitis who was intubated and being ambu-bagged, but death seemed inevitable. Samuel had decided not to use the ventilator. It was a somber moment in an otherwise happy afternoon.

Will's careful planning for the party menu included pre-ordering special hot dogs which almost resembled American style dogs from the Himalaya Coffee store. There was potato salad, cole slaw, corn on the cob, corn bread, a three-bean salad like my mother used to make and soft drinks. Followed by apple pie and ice cream. O Heaven. After the meal, I got out the trumpet and played patriotic songs, blowing so loud my face turned red. Sure enough, within fifteen minutes about forty Nepali kids had gathered, standing at a respectful distance, intently watching as the Mission kids played games like the wheel barrow and three-legged race. Then I got the idea to play the Limbo.

Not every one may be familiar with the Limbo dance. It goes along with a catchy little tune by Chubby Checker from the nineteen-fifties. It's the kind of tune the DJ will play for eighth graders at a middle school dance along with the Macarena and the Mexican Hat Dance, but it is also played at weddings. The tune has a feel of calypso. One by one the dancers go under a horizontal pole without touching it, and without leaning forward. The pole is lowered a bit each time through the tune. Dancers are eliminated one by one until a winner is declared. Along the way, each dancer shows off their physique and coordination.

At the party, Will and Barbara held the ends of a long piece of bamboo and lowered it on cue so the kids could go under. We invited the Nepali onlookers to join the fun, and they all ran over gleefully to get in line. There were cheers and laughter, and at the end the kids demanded that we do it again. My lips were getting tired, but I obliged, and again the kids clamored for more. I played it again and again. Then I thought that I was done and the crowd kept limboing on, even though the music had stopped. So, I joined in one more time. The time flew.

It occurred to me that this might be the first time that the local Nepali kids had done the limbo. *Maybe I am committing some sort of cultural pollution. Are there no limits of decency?* I wondered what some future anthropologist would make of it fifty years hence. Somebody would write a doctoral dissertation on the origin of the Limbo cult in Tansen Palpa Nepal. *I hoped they would not be able to trace it back to me!*

After the party I was still humming the tune as I stopped by the Surgical Ward. A woman from the Terai lay in the Critical Ward. She had experienced a febrile episode that caused her thirty-weeks-gestation fetus to die in utero, and then she had a miscarriage with considerable hemorrhaging. She was admitted to Surgical Critical Ward because it had been a home delivery. She was still septic, bacteria in her bloodstream. There was a sudden silence as I switched off the music in my head. Her temperature was one-hundred-and-five Fahrenheit and her pulse was one-hundred-forty beats per minute. The doctors had already taken her to Theater for a Dilation and Curettage to remove any retained parts of the placenta that might be the cause of her sepsis. The doctors, nurses and students were working to transfuse her, treat her for shock, give antibiotics, control her fever, and give support to her young children and husband.

The younger daughter looked like she was about four-years old. I noticed that the girl was sucking her index finger. *The way my own daughter did as a preschooler.* This thought made me look more closely at the woman in the bed. The patient was drenched in sweat, long black hair now a stringy braid, pale, wearing an oxygen mask. *Remembering my own wife when she became a mother, both of us wondering how our lives would change.* This woman's IV included dopamine, a drug to keep her blood pressure from bottoming out. I looked at the husband, standing still as the activity swirled around him, wondered what he was thinking. The girl sucking her finger clung to his trouser leg and shyly turned her head away when she noticed that I was looking. The team was doing everything they could from what I could tell. *Nothing I can add here.*

I went back to my apartment. It was getting dark as I picked my way down the path by the light of the torch. I considered the ways you can say goodbye in a marriage. *I said my good byes one way, the husband of this patient was saying goodbye in another. I could not decide which was better.* I finally concluded that neither way was very good, each came with its own pain. There were no snakes on the path. I studied my Nepali, wrote in my diary, and went to bed.

In the morning I stopped by Surgical on my way to Pediatrics. The Critical Ward smelled of bleach. The bed which had been the center of attention was empty now; the mattress was bare with a small pile of neatly-folded blue sheets waiting to be spread out for the next occupant after the place had aired out a bit. I looked in the census book. She died at eleven-thirty. She was twenty-seven-years old.

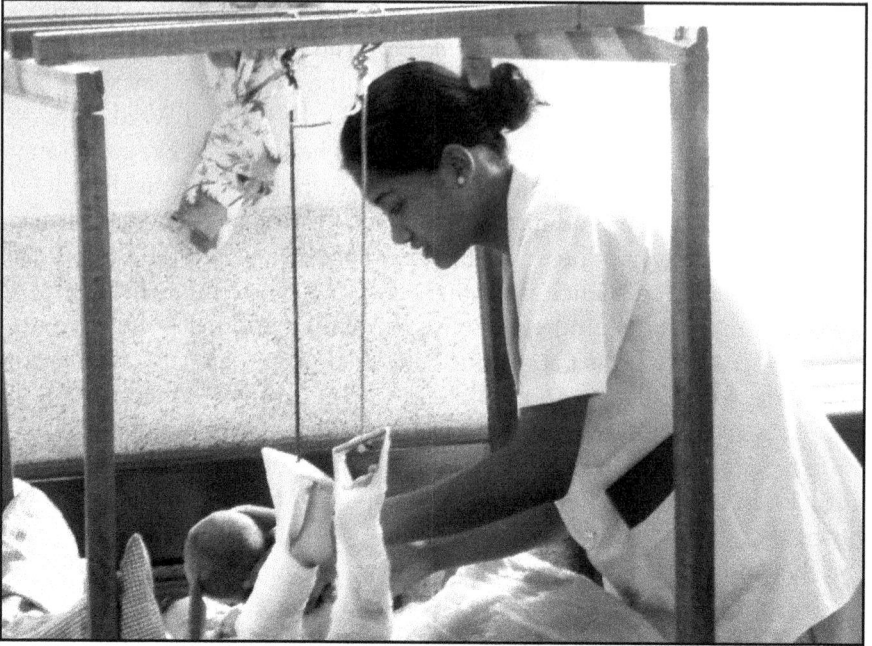

Nurse adjusting "Gallows Traction" on Pediatrics. The child's weight is used to provide counter-traction

Rati Asks for a Favor

Pediatrics at Mission Hospital encompasses a large ward, nearly a third of the total beds. For each patient there is at least one family member, which means that when we have fifty patients there are one hundred people total. At night the mother would sleep under the child's bed or even in the bed with the child. To that number add the ten students, the six staff nurses, and twenty doctors split up into three teams in the morning making rounds. The community outreach people arrive to meet with the patients who need nutritional referrals. There are also food servers from the hospital canteen, cleaning people, a chaplain and people from the supply department or pharmacy delivering equipment and supplies. In other words, about one-hundred-thirty children, family and workers spread out over a floor space roughly equivalent to a tennis court. The net effect was chaos – the "Bus Station Effect" once again. As I walked up the ramp each day, I took time to calm myself – still talking with Little Joe. A short pause to survey the scene, and then dive in.

Despite that initial appearance of chaos, there is a routine to the daily life of the Pediatric Ward. Against this backdrop many individual dramas are being played out, and what I am describing here is only a portion. Like their counterparts in the West, the Nepali nurses have a system to keep track of where everyone is going and what they are doing. Within a few days I was learning the routine and more able to coordinate my activities to be part of the team.

After a couple of days on Pediatrics, Sanjita took me aside for another quick conference with Rati, who had a request. Rati was the faculty member in charge of the second-year curriculum, and she taught obstetrics. She was light-complexioned compared to most Nepalis, and had a smile that made me think of Jackie Kennedy Onassis. Rati was from eastern Nepal and had come to Tansen specifically for this teaching job. I noticed her at Hebron Church earlier in the summer when she arrived in the company of a teenage girl whom I assumed was her daughter. Later I learned that this was the daughter of a friend. Rati was about thirty and unmarried, which was unusual. Most women were married by that age. Rati needed to schedule a day to meet with the first-year students regarding their transition into the second year. Sanjita could float up to Maternity for a day while I would handle the student group by myself. Would I mind terribly? This time Rati did not flutter her eyebrows. Instead, she tilted her gaze so that I could admire her dimples and the graceful arch of her neck. *She needed me to cooperate.* She was also just a bit nervous around me.

In practical terms, to cover Pediatrics by myself meant a lot more work and responsibility for me. I was always there at six in the morning to review all the charts so that I would know some of the patient information in advance. Report was in a mix of Nepali and English and if I did not have a head start I could get lost. I would listen to report with everyone else. After that I would often accompany the pediatricians on physician rounds, and then slip over to the surgical side so I could especially focus on dressing changes. With Sanjita away, I would now be spending less time with the docs, and instead I would observe the students do their structured patient interviews and teaching plans and evaluate their paperwork. I would also devote two hours or more around noon to go with one of the students while she prepared the medications for about ten patients on the medical side. Most of the medications to administer would be antibiotics. Patients on this side were being cared for by the pediatricians as opposed to the surgeons or ortho team.

One of our patients was a skinny little boy who was constipated. He had a "worm impaction." There were so many intestinal parasites in this boy that he was unable to move his bowels and his belly was swollen as if he had a football under the hospital gown. Norma ordered daily enemas until the constipation was relieved. He improved. He was put on a daily dose of worm medication.

On Pediatrics there was one six-bed room just for children in Bryant's Traction, also known as Gallows Traction. When a bone in the leg is broken, muscle spasms will pull it out of alignment, and traction is a way to promote alignment while the bone heals. Nowadays, in the US, the trend is to use hardware on the bone instead, but we still used orthopedic traction in Nepal. In an adult, you also need "counter-traction" to prevent the person in traction from sliding off the end of the bed. But when the patient is small, the child's body becomes the counter-traction; in other words, the traction is balanced so that their legs are pointing straight into the air. Patients with this style of traction always reminded me of hunks of sausage hanging in the window of a market.

One day we took care of a child who was two months old, admitted with a fractured femur. My first question was, "How the heck does a kid that young break their leg?" I immediately thought of child abuse. The answer was, the baby was asleep on mom's back tied in a shawl while mom was out collecting fodder for the goats from grass on a steep slope. The shawl had gotten loose. The baby had tumbled fifty feet down hill. It was lucky to be alive. I could picture the knot coming loose because plenty of mothers used a particular way to tie the shawl when they carried their babies on their backs. One day while walking through the

Outpatient Clinic waiting area I saw the technique for tying it when the mother was by herself. First, the mom bends over so the back is flat. Next, put the baby there, belly down. Momentarily let go while the baby just balances by itself, then flip the shawl over and tie the corners. In Outpatient, I saw a mom do this with a baby that was less than a week old, which amazed me.

When Rati asked me about floating Sanjita, I told her I would take the group by myself for that day as long as Sanjita would be available to come back down to Pediatrics if a problem arose. I tried to bring up the subject of not really liking Pediatrics, but Rati quickly changed the topic, giving words of encouragement. She needed the coverage that day and was not going to get off track.

My first day of supervising the clinical group by myself was without incident. By this time the students were doing better with dressings, and the patients were not being terrorized as much. The staff had gotten to know me a bit better. That day the patients seemed stable and we were not interrupted by any specific emergencies.

One patient who persists in memory from that day was an eleven-year-old boy on the surgical side of Pediatrics. This boy had originally started walking with a limp and complained of leg pain. That was three months earlier. The diagnosis at that time was osteo- sarcoma, a form of bone cancer that shows up in adolescents. The family had been clearly told what would happen if they did not bring him to the hospital two-hundred miles away where we sent our cancer victims. Turned out the family could not afford to send him that far away, or maybe they could not take the time to send a relative with him. So, nothing was done and the cancer grew. In the bed he weighed about sixty pounds. He was all skin and bones. His face was gaunt and the cheeks were drawn in. It hurt to move and he lay in pain. He was to be on the Pediatric Ward for the next week or more while they decided what to do with him. Surgery and chemotherapy were no longer an option. This eleven year old was going to die. The family sat by his bedside in a quiet vigil.

The focus for me that day was to watch one of the students give meds to children for the first time without making any mistakes. Before giving any medications, the student needed to do all the calculations and show their math to the faculty. This was just the same way we did it where I taught in Hawaii. As in the US, some students are better at math than others. Fortunately I directed the student to start the process well in advance. It ended up taking the student more than ninety minutes to do the math, and half of it was wrong. I showed her which ones to re-do, and she asked her fellow students to help her as well. In fairness, I was later to see that most of the other students were very quick and accurate, but on this day, the one I was with was not very confident.

The charge nurse took me aside to tell me that she would be there to start IVs or to re-start them if there was a problem. I think she was worried I might try to do a skill that she had not seen me do, but in fact I was relieved at this. Kids have small veins and I was out of practice. A person needs constant practice to maintain their skill, and we both knew that I had not done this lately. On the other hand, she was as skilled as any nurses I knew from the US. I told her that was fine by me, I was glad to have some backup.

Mission Hospital does not use a unit dose system for IV meds. A battered steel tray with about ten dividers is set out, and into each space a slip of paper with a bed number is placed. As each medication is drawn up, the syringe is put in the bin for that bed number. None of the syringes are actually labeled. After all the meds for about a dozen patients are ready, the whole tray is taken out to the room along with a pile of the medication administration sheets.

To give the medications to the patients, the nurse goes from one bed to the next with the tray and the med charts. There are no trips back to the nurse's station between patients. Just about everything is given IV push, and if the student is nervous it is pushed in faster. A patient's veins can be ruined if the med is given too quickly. When the students give the meds, I find myself saying, *"Bistarai! Bistarai!"* ("Slowly, slowly!") each time, until the student gets a feel for the rate of administration.

We continued to do dressing changes. A sample list of dressings would be:

Ramesh, a young boy who might be seven, but might be six or eight. He looks normal until you unwrapped the dressing from his shin, to reveal the area of exposed shin bone about six inches long. The bone was shiny like a piano key. His marrow had been replaced by cheesy TB material and the orthopedic surgeons had drilled holes in the bone to let it weep out. We did not know whether he would keep the leg. Ramesh never complained and he used a walker to bring himself to the treatment room.

A three-year-old with scalp boils that had been lanced. There were five separate areas to wash, then cover with gauze, and then wrap a gauze turban on his head. Squirmy.

The baby with the leg burns and no toes. Kusmati got premedicated using the ketamine protocol, but still showed signs of terror as she cried.

The other girl with the burns to her legs and buttocks. She was a lot further along in the healing process than Kusmati, and might be going home soon.

154

Gita, a twelve-year-old girl with Cerebral Palsy. Because of her physical handicap, her mother left her for long periods of time lying on a bed of straw in a shed used by animals. When she was admitted, one ear was necrotic and was infested by maggots that looked like short white wiggling rice kernels. Gita had a huge bedsore on her sacrum and was malnourished, weighing only sixty pounds. She was spoon-fed extra Sarbotham Pitto every day, and the surgeons performed a skin flap, rotating the tissue so that the open wound on her sacrum would be covered.

Akash, the baby with the burned head. Another person premedicated using the ketamine protocol.

Abdominal incision on a boy with appendectomy. Corrugated drain in place, sticking out of the wound. We had to be careful not to inadvertently pull the drain out of place when we removed the dressing.

Three elbow dressings of supracondylar fractures that had been surgically repaired. Kids who fell out of trees. This involved removing the arm sling, and it was inevitable that the elbow would wiggle a bit, which caused pain.

Pin care on three children whose leg fractures were being stabilized with K-wires and traction. Because of the traction, these treatments were to be done out in the area where the beds were, not in the treatment room.

The students were improving their skills with each day. I noticed that they did not talk much to the children when they did each dressing change. I told them to talk during the dressing change, and after they were done, to continue talking. Always praise the child for how brave they were, even if the child had cried.

The literal word for "Brave" in Nepali is "*Bahadur*," and it has a special meaning, since so many of our local Nepalis were of the Chhetri caste. The Chhetris are the warrior caste that had settled in Nepal centuries ago. Instead of calling themselves "Chhetri" they will use "*Bahadur*" as their caste name, sometimes abbreviated in writing as "*Bdr.*" It seemed that the patients liked being reminded of their warrior heritage. The students adopted this quickly, and did a better job comforting their small patients after each dressing change. The students themselves were "*bahadur*" as well.

Al was now on the Medical Team. At dinner he told me about a case of attempted suicide using pesticide – an organophosphate overdose. Organophosphate is the general name for weed killer. The rice farmers usually have a can or two around, and drinking it is a popular local way to commit suicide, referred to as "the cuckold's poison," because it was a cure for unrequited love. Unfortunately, weed killer will not kill people as quickly as it works on the weeds. This lady was taking a few days to die while her liver failed. The woman was forty years old. Organophosphates cause a river of tears and a torrent of saliva along with bouts of diarrhea. To reverse these we were giving her a medicine called "PoM" as well as atropine. The cumulative dose of atropine in the past few days was about a hundred milligrams – a staggering amount. She was still failing. She slipped into a coma and died a few days later.

In another bed on Medical was a thirty-year-old woman admitted with sepsis and pneumonia. She was an achondroplastic dwarf, about the height of a three year old child if she could have stood up. She could not walk. At home she slept on a bed of straw in a stable, not in the house with her family. Her scalp was thin and she was covered with some kind of sores which were infected. The doctors thought it was psoriasis but nobody was certain. They were applying silvadene cream to her skin and scalp and she had a striking appearance because she had been slathered in white goo – all but her two eyes which were sticking out. When she spoke you noticed the spaces between her teeth like a picket fence.

The subject of Ova and Parasites came up next. I told them about the child with the worm impaction, and the other child with the "zoo." One of the American medical students proposed a theory that medically-induced tapeworm was bound to become popular as a weight loss modality; it was just a matter of time. After all, it is painless, you can eat all you want and still lose weight, and when you were happy with the results, you could kill the tapeworm with worm medicine. And, no external scars.

Al was quick to share his insight. "There probably are women in Hollywood who will pay ten thousand dollars for something available free right here in rural Nepal." I chimed in to say I wanted to avoid inadvertently smuggling some back into the US.

Someone at the table had read about the Guinea Worm, possibly the most disgusting parasite in the world. We got a graphic description. Thank God there were no Guinea Worms in Nepal.

Photo next page: Akash, the boy with the scalp burn. Taken several weeks after the injury, and the first- and second-degree burns on this face were healing. This is the photo taken by "Padma;" one of the very few photos that has me in it.

Baptism by Fire

Shortly after the July Fourth party, an eight-month-old baby boy was admitted to Pediatrics with an eight percent burn on his left arm, face and scalp. He had been sitting on the floor when a kerosene lamp flashed. It was fueled by kerosene all right, but not like an American hurricane lamp with glass and a wick and a handle. In the rural areas of the Palpa district the houses had no electricity and they used kerosene to light the night. It may have been a simple tin can with some holes cut in the top with a cotton wick stuck in one of the holes, more like a Molotov cocktail that had not been thrown. His name was Akash.

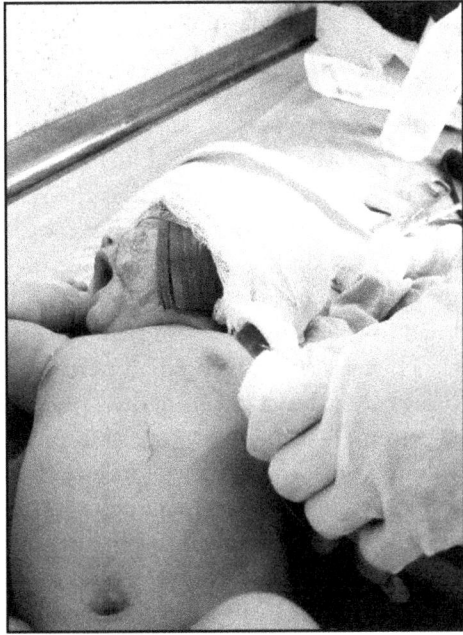

When I saw him he had an IV in the good arm. Gauze was wrapped around the burned arm and his hand. His head was swaddled like a turban, and you could see that his face was burned on the left side just about to the nose. I bent over closely and used the torch to look at his eyelids and eyes. The left eyelid was swollen shut and the eyelashes had been singed, but otherwise they seemed undamaged. The doctors asked us to unwrap the bandage at morning rounds and they would return when it was off. We briefly studied the drawing of the wound that the ER staff put in the medical record, and then we removed the bandages, slowly and carefully. First the gauze, then the banana leaf. We then irrigated with saline to gently wash the silvadene from the wound.

His hand was burned, mostly second degree with huge blisters, and seemed painful but he actually tolerated it better than I thought he might when we wrapped it and splinted it. He could move his fingers and elbow. The head bandage was off now. I took out my torch to see his scalp. The boy's left ear was chalky white. Eschar. It was going to slough off completely. Probably within a few days at most. It was so fragile I thought *I might be able to scrape it off with a tongue blade.* Not that I would even try, but I thought to myself *I bet I could.* Akash would not have an ear when the dead tissue was done sloughing off. Just a hole in the side of his head that he could hear through. His ear hole was not bleeding but it was gummed up with silvadene, the antiseptic cream used to prevent infection.

There were two sections of scalp in which the skin had turned a peculiar leathery color: sort of translucent and crusty, like you would find on a roast pig that had just been served at a *luau*. This was also eschar. A full thickness burn to the scalp. The dead tissue was still covering his skull, but when that too sloughed off, he would have two areas on his skull, each about three inches in diameter, where there was not even any periosteum – the wound in these spots had gone right down to the bone.

This was a relatively small percentage of burn, but very serious. Early in my career I worked in neurosurgical ICU, and I knew that it would be extremely difficult to graft skin onto the area where the bone showed. A graft needs a blood supply. Here there would be no opportunity to develop capillary buds from below a proposed graft, and the adjacent areas of skin would need to heal before flapping could be done. Even in the US this would have been difficult.

By this time I was getting better at holding it together emotionally when I was working with the burn wounds. I was able to look at this child without having a visceral response. In my mind I scrolled through various burn wounds I had seen or heard about, and calculated the odds of survival based on the severity. From a scientific perspective, this kid was in deep trouble and this would all unfold in slow motion over a period of days or weeks. *I can see this one coming. And it is going to suck. In a big way.*

The surgeon came to the room where the crib was. It was one of the Nepali surgeons, a soft-spoken and kindly man who was well respected for his competence and work ethic. The student held the torch as he looked at the scalp very quietly, and turned the baby's head to see all sides. He looked in Akash's ear. He turned to us and indicated we should put the new dressing on.

The surgeon sat on the low wooden stool, near the mother, and started to talk. In Nepali, he told the mother what he thought about the boy's chances. It was pretty much the same as I expected. I could not make it all out exactly but I could tell by the way the mother reacted that it was not good news. We would do all we could but the child was probably going to die. I followed him out after he was done talking, to make sure I heard him correctly.

Mom was doing okay until then but had a major crying spell and buried her face in her hands. Now she sat on the small wooden stool by the bedside as the nurses comforted her. My own Nepali language skills were not good enough to help her, but suffering is a universal language and I could see how badly she was taking it. As the nurses comforted her, the student and I re-wrapped the baby's dressings while he lay on the crib.

The baby cried and his mom came over to the bedside. She seemed reluctant to touch him, as if he might break. I thought to myself, *No matter how sick, this kid needs his mother's love. She has held him until now.* I told the student to tell her, "You can pick Akash up and hold him as much as you want. He does not have to lie in the crib all the time." She sat on the little stool and we showed her how to hold him so she would not squeeze his burned arm under the gauze. She held him, fumbling at first. He rooted around for her breast and she offered it to him, reaching under her blouse. She rocked him as he sucked. I could see her holding him gently and gazing into his eyes as she fed him. *How many times has she looked at him that way,* I thought. *She may not be holding him much longer.* The nurse stood at her side, with one hand on the mom's shoulder. I wondered what was going through the mom's mind at that moment. *I wonder how many more times she will pick him up.* I could see the mom was still red-eyed. Her tears fell on the baby. I decided to check on my other students and left the room.

The next day the boy was still there. The child was surprisingly vigorous despite his injury. The surgeons were going to wait a few days before debriding the scalp wound. Debriding is the medical term for removal of dead tissue and cleaning the wound edges until only living tissue remains. Because the surgeons knew it would expose the bone they were cautious. The student and I changed the dressing. I mentioned this case to Samuel, the pediatrician. Because the child was admitted by the surgeons, Samuel did not automatically examine him or write orders at first; but now Samuel went over to take a look and to order some different antibiotics. Samuel was going to give this baby boy every chance.

The mom seemed withdrawn. She was helpless so we told her there was one thing she could do: since she was breastfeeding him, he needed nourishment in order to survive. We told her that she herself needed to increase her protein intake and eat more so she could produce the best possible milk. She seemed really encouraged by this. In fact, the boy was sucking hungrily. So from then on, we saw her coaxing him to suck more, and she herself started eating meat and yogurt. I suppose that in the US, he would have been moved to a formula supplement, but here that was not something we did.

The day came for the first debridement, which would be performed by the surgeons under anesthesia in Theater. It was a relief because that meant we did not have to do the dressing that day. The next day, after the debridement, we saw that his burned outer ear had been removed. The skull bone that had been hidden by the leathery eschar was now exposed. It looked as if it was polished ivory right out of a jewelry store window. The texture of it reminded me of a necklace I bought in the *Bajar* that was made of polished yak bone.

For the next few days we now had three major burn dressings on the list. Kusmati, Akash, and the girl whose buttocks were burned. A few mornings later I was in early as usual, and the night nurse told me that one of the burned girls had died.

My heart sank. *Kusmati?*

No, it was the other one, the one whose burn was on the buttocks and which we had difficulty keeping clean. She developed burn sepsis in the middle of the night, spiking a high fever, and died of shock despite efforts to revive her. It was unexpected. *Thank God I was not there when it happened.*

We carried on with the plan for the day.

At the Guest House, there was a Nepali family that lived next door to me. In Honolulu, my apartment is in a quiet residential neighborhood with mostly retirees and there is some distance between houses. By contrast, in the Guest House complex behind the hospital, the apartments were a lot closer together. The father worked in the x-ray department and there were three young children. The oldest was a girl around eight who tended the small garden they planted at the end of the walkway. Next were two boys, six and three years old. The day the baby girl died, I noticed them more than I previously had.

This night, the three children next door seemed to be awake later than usual. They were singing songs. They were laughing and playing. It was some kind of guessing game. I think the older daughter was giving the youngest his bath. He was splashing and squealing with delight. The parents occasionally interjected words to keep on track. As the evening ended, the girl read a long bedtime story out loud. It was in Nepali and I have no idea what it was about, I could just hear it faintly through the window. I fell asleep to the sound of happy joyful children who were having childish fun and who were experiencing the simple delight of being in the world, full of possibility and love.

The Maoists and the Attack on Tansen

The Peace Corps formerly sent volunteers to rural Nepal but suspended operations in Nepal in 1995, after the civil war had been going on for a year or two. In 2001 the royal family was massacred during a dinner at their palace in Kathmandu, and the cremation at

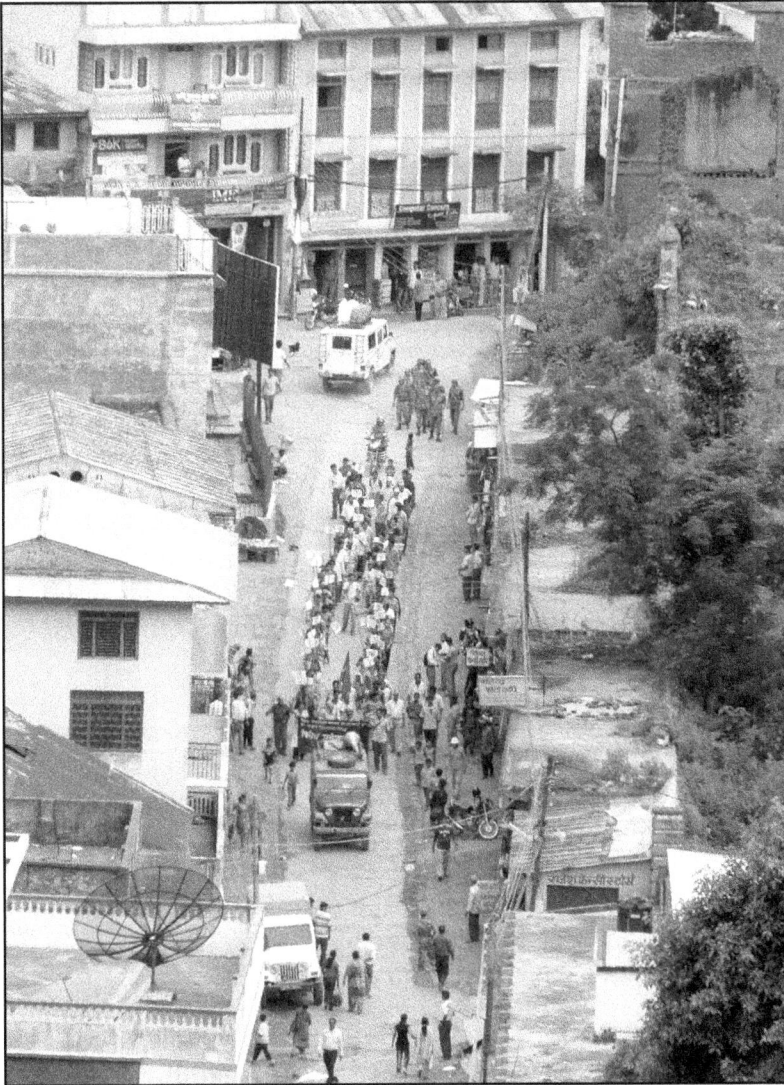

The day of the Maoist rally in downtown Tansen. To the right, ruins of the government building burned in January 2006. At the far end, the internet café. Maoists followed by a small contingent of soldiers.

Pashupattinath was a national spectacle. The King's brother became the new king. He was not popular. The civil war continued until 2006 when the Eight-Party Alliance was formed. I was only vaguely aware of this before I bought my ticket to Tansen.

The day I arrived, the Buck slowed down to pass right through a Maoist rally being held near the bus depot. There were large red banners and people holding loudspeakers. Three-hundred people were in attendance. As they made way for the Buck to pass, they all held their arms with hands clasped, and looked down. I was riveted to the window. I could not figure out what this gesture meant, but it seemed respectful. I was impressed that they all did it on cue as if it were a salute.

During the civil war, the army was authorized to shoot to kill when they met a suspected Maoist. Sanjita told me about the first Maoist she ever met. "This happened when I was a student at TNS. He was a patient, the army had shooted him in the leg." I nodded, deciding not to correct her grammar. "Our teacher told us not to talk with him at all. He was in the men's ward, and guarded by soldiers with orders to kill him if he tried to escape. So during the day we never spoke with him, but since there were three students on night duty, as soon as she left we all went straight to the place in the men's ward where he lay, to talk with him about it and ask him questions." She told me she did a case study on him since it was unusual for Mission Hospital to admit people with gunshot wounds. "He told us about his life and why he was a Maoist. He was from western Nepal and the conditions there were very bad. We all liked him and learned a lot from him."

Armed Maoist rebels attacked Tansen on January 31st, 2006, and I was in Tansen nearly a year and a half after the Maoist attack. Many of the missionaries at Mission Hospital witnessed the events. This is the story as told to me by one of the missionaries that was in Tansen during the attack.

There are three geographical points in Tansen that played a role. The first is Shree Nagar *danda*. (A *danda* is a hill). Tansen is a hill town, nestled halfway up the hill with maybe another five-hundred feet of vertical elevation. The hill is planted with pine trees in an effort to conserve the watershed of the town. Hiking paths crisscross the hill through the foot-deep pine needles on the floor of the forest. From the hill there is a clear view into the town. Gairegau, the neighborhood where the Fourth of July picnic was held, also enjoyed a panoramic view. Homes in this neighborhood are rented out to doctors and missionaries from the hospital. From the porch of each there is a panoramic view. The missionaries viewed the attack from these houses.

Next is the *Tundikhel,* or Parade Ground, a large flat oval space at the foot of the town, big enough to break out a string of ponies and play polo. At the eastern end was the barracks of the army. It was perched on a steep hill for security reasons. The army dug a twenty-foot deep trench across the mid-portion of the Tundikhel as a security measure. A guard tower and barbed wire completed the perimeter.

Third was the Tansen *Durbar,* or palace. The *Durbar* was built in the 1920s, the largest brick building in the Palpa District. The *Durbar* occupied the center of town. A plaza of green space surrounded the *Durbar,* and a brick building housed a dozen soldiers who served as its garrison. One edge of the grounds of the *Durbar* served as the boundary for the *Bajar* of Flat Street. All government business for Palpa district was conducted there.

The armed Maoists approached Tansen on foot from the north, behind Shree Nagar hill. Local people were given a three days' warning that an attack would come. Any merchant with any sense packed up their stuff and hunkered down out of harms way. The army got wind of the impending attack but dismissed it, doing nothing.

The attack was coordinated by rebel leaders from the top of the hill, using cell phones to stay in touch with the different elements of their forces. From the height, they started off with mortar and machine gun fire directed at the army barracks. A part of their forces was used to keep the army bottled up at one end of the *Tundikhel.* The barbed wire and trench that had been intended to keep out a rebel attack, served to prevent the army from making a sortie out of the barracks area, because there was only one exit. The soldiers were bottled up by a smaller force.

The barracks attack was not the main objective, however. Once they diverted the army to dealing with the threat to the barracks, the Maoist forces attacked the *Durbar.* They set it on fire. The soldiers defending it were trapped inside. The *Durbar* burned all night and was gutted. After the attack, a team of soldiers used dogs to sniff out the charred bodies of the defenders.

Sporadic fire went on all night, by morning the Maoist forces had withdrawn. Fourteen army soldiers and an undetermined number of Maoists were killed. No civilians were killed. Some of the missionaries said that later you could see the footprints of the Maoist's boots and it was clear due to the small boot size, that the soldiers had been mostly women and children. The town was deserted for three days.

Later, the Maoists also attacked Butwal, a two-hour drive to the south, in the *Terai.* Butwal was where the road to Tansen intersected with the road that went along the southern border of Nepal through the *Terai.* Theoretically the Maoists could have rolled on through the

Terai, but after the Butwal attack, the Maoists withdrew. They did not gain any territory in the military sense. They had, however, shocked the government by their actions, and shown that the government could not protect itself against armed military action. The psychological impact of this was tremendous and led to renewed pressure on the government to sign a truce.

The hospital was more than a mile away from this activity, and was never under threat. Foreign aid workers were never involved. But the anxiety level went up, and the hospital spent time to develop a plan for evacuation of foreign workers if that should ever become necessary. The attack produced a chilling effect on morale among foreign aid workers and their willingness to go to Tansen. For the record, no foreign aid worker was ever targeted by the Maoists, not in Tansen, not anywhere.

I did not know of the attack until after I had agreed to go there. One time I was walking with Ellie on a road that skirted the hill, looking down on a cricket game taking place on the *Tundikhel*. We could hear the crack of the bat even from this distance. He pointed out the stripe of dirt that extended across the grass, cutting the *Tundhikel* in two. It marked the location of the trench, now filled in since the peace agreement.

He said, "Filling in the trench is a visible mark of progress I had not expected to see in my life time. We can make peace. Things are much better here."

The *Durbar* was still there. Or at least, the remains of it were. The walls still stood but the roof was open to the sky. There were piles of bricks nearby. The doors were boarded up. It was a ruin.

There were about a hundred soldiers in the Tansen garrison that summer. In the mornings they would run past the hospital wearing matching track suits, and climb to the top of Shree Nagar Hill to the Buddhist shrine. They would march on the *Tundikhel* every afternoon and play soccer or volleyball. Late in the afternoon they would patrol through the *Bajar*. Twenty guys in fatigues would stroll purposefully in single file, each carrying a four-foot long bamboo *lathi*, like a drill team. One afternoon I watched them from the shady side of Flat Street, where I leaned against the door jamb of a small shop, with my camera around my neck. The sergeant noticed me, the only *videshi*, and hurried over.

He told me, "No photo! No photo!"

I put the camera in my pocket, saying, "*Thik cha!*" I did not want my camera confiscated.

One Saturday in early July before the rains came, the early morning heat shimmered as a green jeep with a huge loudspeaker came slowly through the hospital neighborhood, blaring. I could not make out what they were saying, and asked a shop owner to help me and translate. He shook his head and told me that the Maoists would hold a rally that afternoon. There would be a *bandh* all day – the shops in the *Bajar* would stay closed until the rally was over.

The rally itself was a sort of parade along Flat Street. First, the loudspeaker jeep with traditional Nepali music blaring followed by people carrying large red flags. Then, about a hundred people marching solemnly behind. A contingent of twenty army soldiers followed a short distance after them. The soldiers marched smartly in step with their *lathis*. There were no firearms in sight that day, and the event was peaceful.

The Maoist rally made me think back to Memorial Day parades in small-town New England and I thought, *they sure could use a high school band and some majorettes to liven this up, or throw some candy.* Actually, there were few spectators. The shops opened about an hour after the rally ended.

Of all the shops in the *Bajar*, there was only one where the prices were posted, western-style, for all to see. No bargaining necessary. It was run by a Nepali man who attended the Christian church. The Himalaya Coffee shop specialized in Western-style foods with western brand names, such as Heinz Ketchup, Mayonnaise, Kellogg's Cereal or tuna fish. It was the place to obtain Cadbury's chocolate, or Pringle's potato chips. Or Pepsi, or a six-pack of beer. Even though Bimla did my shopping, I always stopped in at Himalaya Coffee if only to look at what they had on the shelves. Often I would run into other missionaries there, and it seemed as though I was always running into two women from a Danish NGO who were based here in Tansen working on nutrition issues. To browse there was a comfortable reminder of western-style shopping.

One evening at the *Bajar* I stopped at Himalaya Coffee to buy ketchup. As I left the store, I saw a jeep pull up with four soldiers carrying machine pistols – the kind the Israeli army is often pictured with. Mean little weapons that can spray bullets like a garden hose. This kind of gun is not very accurate but sure to splash everything in range. The green paint was peeling off these weapons but the underlying metal was shiny. I decided to move along, because the soldiers seemed edgy. I put my camera out of sight. *If they were worried about trouble, I did not need to be there.* I walked up Flat Street to Nanglo's. I looked at the vegetable sellers on the stone gazebo outside Nanglo's just to see what they had, even though I did not buy any produce.

As I stood there, the same army jeep pulled up to the front of the restaurant. The soldiers quickly fanned in different directions, taking up positions in the corners of the square and on top of the gazebo there. Behind them, a black SUV pulled up. Out stepped a muscular man wearing new blue jeans, a gold wristwatch, a dress shirt and pointy leather cowboy boots. His hair was short but oiled and slicked back. He turned to help a woman out of the vehicle behind him. She was about his age, wearing a low cut red gown that looked like a prom dress. She carried a small purse and wore a glittery necklace. Evidently I was watching the local military commander on a date with his wife. His security guards seemed to be settling in for the evening. I decided to walk back to the hospital compound and headed off toward the Jerusalem Tunnel.

I learned later that the main Maoist leader in town was a *hotel-wallah* - a small business owner who did a lot of contract work with the hospital. He had been around the hospital all summer. He seemed to be a sort of middleman for many of the relatives of patients - organizing transportation, loaning money, and advocating for them. It finally dawned on me that this was all part of his political work, so I asked the hospital Chaplain to introduce me to him. The Chaplain brought me to him and we shook hands a week before I left. The Maoist leader was a pleasant potbellied guy with a wispy beard who always wore a hat to cover his bald spot. Like the soldiers, he would not allow me to take his picture. And now I knew one more reason why the Maoists would never attack the hospital. Their leader depended on the hospital for his livelihood. If the hospital had been damaged, his hotel would lose all its guests.

The night of the rally, Padma told us a story she heard from Barbara. Two years before their first child was born, Ellie and Barbara were in Somalia working for a Christian NGO there. They lived in a rural area, providing basic medical care. The NGO that sponsored them provided a station wagon, the only vehicle in the village. One night, six armed men came to the house. Barbara hid in a closet before they knew she was there. Ellie was kidnapped at gunpoint and Barbara thought she would never see him again. She cried and prayed for six hours. *Barbara, who could work with burn victims all day and not lose her sense of optimism and hope. Barbara, who knew when and how to enjoy a beer in a proper pub.* This was new insight about Barbara and it took a minute to sink in.

Ellie returned in the morning, unhurt. Turns out the gunmen were not political. They only wanted the car and did not wish to kill the missionary. Ellie and Barbara decided to leave Somalia. Ellie never spoke of this incident.

Visitors From Kathmandu

In July I was spending every day on Pediatrics and getting to know the students and staff better. I was focusing on the task at hand despite my reaction to the terrible problems that patients came with. The next time the Buck returned from Kathmandu we all met Pastor Matt and his family. They stayed three days and would be driving back with a doctor who was going on vacation. For the past five years, they had been based in Kathmandu. Matt spoke with a Scottish brogue and a baritone voice. Matt used the term "aye" in conversation, which caught my ear since it resembled the way a Mainer would say "ayuh."

That evening some of the medical staff joined us at the Guest House, to receive our visitors in style. At dinner the talk turned to the driving habits of people in Kathmandu. In Nepal, traffic goes on the left, which is confusing enough for an American. Beyond this, we all agreed that there seemed to be no rules. There are at least five ways to honk your horn in Nepal, sometimes it meant – "Go ahead of me," and sometimes it meant – "Stop what you are doing." Sometimes a horn did not seem to mean anything at all. The big *Tata* trucks sported multi-tone horns that reminded me of a Schoenberg tone row when they were sounded, and I wondered why nobody bothered to program the horn to play an actual tune. Everyone at the table had a story or two about the near-miss traffic accidents they had seen.

We were incredulous to learn that Matt and his wife had each failed the Nepali motorcycle license practical exam the first time around. Surely, this was impossible given the death-defying habits of the Nepali drivers we had seen. Matt said he failed because he assumed the test should be done at the usual motorcycle speed that would have been used in London. In Nepal, the test was to see how slowly you could drive in close traffic without hitting anything.

You could flunk your automobile test if you left your headlights on. At this, Al said, "Maybe that's because they know that electrical power is so expensive in this country and they want to conserve energy." This was typical of Al's perspective on life in Nepal.

Our guests also told us about buying fresh meat in Kathmandu. They no longer ate pork, they said. It was because one day she returned from the market, put the pork roast on the cutting board, and realized that it was still wiggling due to the worms. The roast moved about an inch along the counter in just a minute or two as she watched. We were eating meat loaf that evening, made from Buff. Al brought up the idea of tapeworm-induced weight loss.

Will Masters was sitting further down the table and I thought he had not been listening, but he waved one finger in the air while he used the napkin on his lip, chewed a bit, and finished swallowing. "The life cycle of tapeworm is a bit more complicated than that, I am afraid. If you ingest the worm in its egg form, as opposed to a larvae, you may find that you develop onchocercosis, a full grown worm crawling around inside your skull." We looked at him in admiration. He did not often eat with us, but Will was surely elevating the caliber of dinner talk. He continued, "These can only be removed by a neurosurgeon. Tapeworm can also cause a type of abdominal growth called a hydatid cyst, which is fatal to eighty percent of patients if it is untreated." *So much for that idea.*

I decided not to eat any more pork for the rest of the summer.

Matt described his job as the missionaries minister. In this capacity he traveled throughout Nepal from his base in the capital. Most often the local church services in English were run by the missionaries themselves. Matt would be here to meet with the prayer groups, give support to the missionaries, and provide a Eucharistic service. At Mission Hospital four or five of the long term missionaries were preparing to go back to the sending country within the next six months. One evening, Matt led a men's group on the subject of re-integrating into society. He used his laptop to pull out some references to Philip to use as an example. Matt's main point was to discuss where you go from here. What is your career after this? Do you ever stop being a missionary? What is normal life after this?

Far and away the highlight of Matt's visit was the Eucharistic service at which bread and grape juice would be consecrated. For this, all the *videshis* came. The children left while the adults listened to the sermon. The first part was on steeling yourself from sin as defined in the Ten Commandments, so as not to go to hell when you die. *Not exactly on my front burner of issues.*

I found myself thinking; *at least he's getting beyond Acts.* This is the favorite section of the Bible for all missionaries. At all the prayer activities it seemed as though we were with The Apostle Paul on the three voyages, over and over. I had been thinking *if we get on the boat with Paul one more time I am going to get seasick.*

Then Matt turned to the topic of letting God be in control. "God," he said, "would have a plan for you that could only be shared on a "need to know" basis. You would not be allowed to see the far end of the plan until you bought into the close end, and in the meantime, you needed to stick closer to God at each junction in your life while the directions were being sorted out." *That's me all right.*

Missionaries sing more fervently than any other group of Christians, and as we shared the bread and grape juice, the hymn was *Be Thou My Vision*. It seemed to be more beautiful than I remembered it, as if I had never really heard the words before.

> *Be Thou my Vision, O Lord of my heart;*
> *Naught be all else to me, save that Thou art.*
> *Thou my best Thought, by day or by night,*
> *Waking or sleeping, Thy presence my light.*
> *Be Thou my Wisdom, and Thou my true Word;*
> *I ever with Thee and Thou with me, Lord;*
> *Thou my great Father, I Thy true son;*
> *Thou in me dwelling, and I with Thee one.*
> *Be Thou my battle Shield, Sword for the fight;*
> *Be Thou my Dignity, Thou my Delight;*
> *Thou my soul's Shelter, Thou my high Tower:*
> *Raise Thou me heavenward, O Power of my power.*
> *Riches I heed not, nor man's empty praise,*
> *Thou mine Inheritance, now and always:*
> *Thou and Thou only, first in my heart,*
> *High King of Heaven, my Treasure Thou art.*
> *High King of Heaven, my victory won,*
> *May I reach Heaven's joys, O bright Heaven's Sun!*
> *Heart of my own heart, whatever befall,*
> *Still be my Vision, O Ruler of all.*

If it was only that simple, I thought to myself.

After the service, we had a wonderful fried chicken dinner with mashed potatoes and gravy. As we ate I found myself humming the last hymn and looking at the lyrics on the program so I could recall them. I was to leave for Pokhara the next day, so I spent some time getting last minute advice, then went back to the apartment to prepare. I would be traveling lightly, just my day pack. I double and triple checked my passport – after all, getting the visa extended was the purpose of going to Pokhara, and I did not want to forget this document. I dug out the ATM card from my suitcase and put it with the passport as well. This would be my first chance to see if the card worked in Nepal. I figured I would need another ten thousand rupees to get through the summer.

Trip to Pokhara

My sixty-day visa to Nepal would expire July twentieth so I always knew I would need to officially extend my stay with a little stamp on the passport. I could go to Pokhara or to Kathmandu to renew it by paying the fee at the government office. Pokhara is seven hours away by bus, along a winding mountain road. It is the favorite spot for UMN people to go when they needed a break from Tansen. The highlight of Pokhara is the Phewa Taal, one of the few large lakes in the country. On a good day, Fishtail Peak and the nearest mountains of the Himalayas are reflected in the lake surface. A popular activity is to hire a rowboat and float around. Pokhara is a popular tourist town and the starting point for the Annapurna trek, one of the spectacular outdoor experiences of the world. Tourists can also sign on for side trips to go river rafting or wildlife viewing. The tourist hotels are clustered near Phewa Taal in the Lakeside district, a pleasant little bubble. The slogan was, "You can't come to Nepal and not see Pokhara."

Many of the *videshis* were planning to take their families to Pokhara the week of the sixteenth and they chartered a special bus so they could go as a group. *What was the point of that?* I wondered. If I was going to Pokhara to "get out of Dodge," it would be better to spend the time by myself instead of with the same exact group of people that I saw in Tansen every day. I figured I should go before then. The government visa offices were only open on weekdays, another factor to consider.

It was raining heavily as I walked from the Guest House, through the hospital, out the door, and about a mile to the depot. My glasses fogged and I rolled up my pant legs so they would not get muddy. I looked down and realized that my tan from Hawaii was completely gone, my legs were white. My umbrella did not protect me from the wind. The bus depot was a large concrete plaza lined with small restaurants and hotels at the foot of Steep Street in the lower part of town. I rarely went there. It occurred to me that I should have planned this better since I did not know exactly when the bus was to leave. For that matter I did not know where to get the ticket. I would have to ask. While I walked I turned over in my head the words for ticket, bus, and price.

At first I mistook the Police office for the ticket booth, because it was very official looking. The sergeant stepped out on the porch with me to point me in the right direction, and I crossed the plaza again rehearsing the words. It was an easy task to buy the ticket and it only cost a hundred sixty rupees. Now I had an hour to wait. I went to a small restaurant that had a "*momo*" sign and ordered a plate of *buff momo* along with a lemon soda. *Momo* is a Tibetan dish but it is widely available since it is popular. Each *momo* is a small piece of meat wrapped in dough like a Pierogi or ravioli. The restaurant was a dark, windowless place lit by a bare bulb and it smelled of grease. On the walls were old movie posters and cigarette ads, a bit grimy. I could smell the cooking oil that sizzled behind the counter. I sat on a wooden bench behind a wooden table. A young man with a week's growth of beard sat opposite me without asking permission. *Namaste.* His hands were dirty and he smelled of alcohol. His eyes were bloodshot. He seemed to already know that I worked at the hospital. "I am a small man!" he kept repeating. "I have brothers and sisters that need to go to school." He asked me for money. I looked at him but did not smile. I tried to ignore him as I dipped my *momo* in the *achaar*, which was a bit peppery. He kept talking. When I was finished eating I got up to pay at the counter, brushing past him wordlessly. "I am a small man!" He followed me into the rain for a bit then gave up since he had no umbrella. I walked across the depot to the ticket seller's booth. The young man working there invited me to take a seat behind the counter with him. There was a huge bale of *Sal* leaves bundled up, the kind the Nepalis stitch together to make disposable plates, ready to be shipped off somewhere.

The Pokhara bus came right on time. It was old with ripped upholstery and small seats. There was the usual little plastic glow-in-the-dark Ganesh on the dashboard next to the driver. The ceiling of the inside was originally painted with a fanciful design like the Sistine Chapel but was now peeling and I could not quite make out what it represented. I am sure it was beautiful at one time in the past. Because of the rain, nobody was riding on the roof of the bus that day. I got a seat in the back. The other passengers formed a tableau typical of Nepal, with shaven-headed Buddhist nuns, assorted Magars, people with *dokaas* full of produce, families, and the like. We would take a half-hour break for *dal-bhaat* along the way and we expected to reach Pokhara after seven hours on the road.

As the trip went on, I found myself thinking about Celeste and the prayer beads, which were on my desk top in the apartment. I thought about all my attempts to use healthy coping skills while in Nepal. I had not meditated in any kind of Buddhist sense. *Did Celeste really meditate?* Celeste certainly knew she needed to control her anger, which was what had drawn her to the Buddhists in the first place. A day or two before, Celeste sent me an email in which she said she had been arrested for DUI. She gave no details and I tried to picture the possible scene. She never drank with me because she knew I did not drink. She often went out drinking with a couple of girlfriends, so it would have been at night.

I wondered whether she would have tried to flirt with the officer or tried to argue. *When she was sober she could switch back and forth between each strategy with surgical precision.* She was pretty tightly wound and I wondered whether she ever was able to actually get physical with anybody *unless* she had been drinking. *Probably not,* then ruefully *but I was never going to find out.* She was definitely having a different experience than I was this summer.

The bus rocked as it made its way through the winding mountain roads, and it occurred to me that from among a half-million women in Honolulu, I had to be in love with this one. I wondered about her arrest and whether she slept it off in jail. Somehow I was attracted to dysfunctional women, but it was a two-way street – it seemed that they could also spot me a mile away. After the divorce, it was nice to hang out with Celeste, because she was such a fun person to talk with, but she was never going to let it go beyond the level of friends. I loved her or at least I called it love, but it was hard to categorize. Maybe it was mainly because I was lonely and she shared so many attributes, good and bad, with my former wife. *Was it really "love?" Or just holding on to the familiar?* There was a part of Celeste that was always on guard, and I wondered whether Celeste ever truly was able to let somebody past the walls she put up. *How does a person get to that point?* I wanted to know but I would never get close enough to find out. *I would do anything for Celeste, but at the same time I was never going to move on as long as Celeste was there.* I wondered if there were any other men in her life. If there were, she was very, very careful never to share that with me. *I was in Honolulu to run away from my life on the east coast. What was Celeste running away from?*

I would have loved to share Nepal with Celeste, but it was then that I realized that if I was enjoying Nepal at all, it was partly because I was free from that kind of person while I was here. This trip was an experiment to find new aspects of myself. Though it was difficult to get divorced, it was clear to me that it was the right thing to do for my own mental health. As I looked out the window of the bus, I wondered whether now in Honolulu, Celeste was a burden. I could make a fresh start and not have her in my life when I returned to Honolulu. *Why not? I have mojo; I am in charge of my destiny.* I made a note to myself to change my life when I got back. *Hell, it has already changed. There is no return from here.*

The bus came to a place where there were six houses by the side of the road and stopped to let people on. At first I did not notice the man with the goat. Soon there was a small pile of goat pellets on the floor of the bus not far from me. There was a girl about twelve on the seat in front of me. She was wearing a nondescript *lungi* and I did not pay her much attention at first. She got on after the first hour or so, and rode for four hours. This part of the trip was curvy as the road hugged the mountainside. We could look down in to the valley below, shimmering watery paddies full of new rice. The river tumbled down the center of the valley, a ribbon of rocks and whitewater. Flat straight irrigation canals tapped into it every now and again to reroute the water through the paddies with their bow-shaped dikes that looked like fish scales when viewed from this distance. The shoots gave the terraced paddies a brilliant color of electric green. Now and again there would be a house, some with tin roofs others with thatch. I was entranced by the scenery. I stuck my face out the open window so I did not have to smell the goat, and enjoyed the view. If somebody had seen me, I am sure there was a beatific expression on my face. It was all so new and such a pleasant change from Tansen. I had a sense of freedom and felt good that I had found the bus myself. The seat next to the girl ahead was empty so she slept on the seats. I looked at the trucks going by - the most common make of truck is by the Tata Corporation - I laughed when I realized that the word "*tata*" in Nepali alphabet, looked like a crude child's drawing of two sets of wheels. I wondered if that was how the name was chosen. It was a verbal pun and visual that would have made no sense to anybody who only spoke English.

After an hour or two the girl suddenly woke up, popped her head out the window and barfed. The wind pushed the vomit up along the window which was now suddenly opaque, and blew a cloud directly into my face, fogging my glasses and stinging my eyes. She might as well have aimed for me. Whoa! *Did you see what God just did to me?* I thought. My initial surprise and anger melted into laughter as I recalled Hunter S. Thompson and wiped her vomit off my face. *That was rude.* It snapped me out of my reverie.

We were almost through the mountains with about an hour to go. The rain was now stopped but the sky was overcast. The bus braked heavily going down a long hill, because there were logs blocking the road. As the bus stopped, a bunch of guys came out of a small thatched hut to argue with the driver. I thought I saw an assault rifle, but I quickly put my head down, so I could not really tell what was happening. They seemed to be demanding money. *What if they are Maoists?* The driver turned off the engine and the sudden silence fell over everything and everyone. At that moment I felt conspicuous - *the only westerner on the bus*. I sat as low in the seat as I could, and tried not to look. *The only one with blond hair.* After ten minutes, and handing over some cash, the guys moved the logs that had been blocking the road and the bus started up again. I gave a quizzical palms-up-in-the-air gesture - nobody on the bus could speak English, all they said was "*bhandh*" which meant "closed" or "strike." As we rode the rest of the way, the other riders were relaxed again but I never figured out who set up the roadblock or what had happened. Later in Tansen Ellie said he doubted they were Maoists but he could not offer an idea as to what they were about.

The Hotel Barahi

It was hot, muggy and overcast in Pokhara. I found the Lakeside area, where all the hotels and restaurants were located overlooking the water. On the south end of the main drag was a huge tree with dozens of hotel and bar signs nailed to it. There was the Hotel Barahi sign, with an arrow to the right. So I walked down the side street past a small ice cream place. At the entrance to the hotel was a small gatehouse with a uniformed guard and there was a head-high stone wall with broken glass embedded in the top. Shiny nice cars in the parking lot, which was paved. Of all the hotels in the Lakeside district, this one gave a special discount for UMN people which worked out to eight US Dollars a night. I decided to get a basic room and not pay the extra fee for air conditioning.

As I checked in I could see the pool, where some pale Japanese tourists wore sunglasses and lipstick as they lounged in bikinis and read Japanese glamour magazines. *Lipstick? At the pool? What's up with that? Do those tourists actually go in the water?* A small hot tub, giving off steam, was empty. The hotel grounds included some bushes cut like topiary in geometric shapes which seemed foreign to me. The restaurant was right near the check in, there was a bar with gleaming bottles of western liquor, and I could see a buffet table for breakfast. A sign in English indicated that a traditional Nepali music show started at six, featuring dancers in folk costumes. A small group of athletic-looking trekkers from Japan stood in the parking lot, packing their matching duffel bags in to a van taxi. Here at the hotel were more westerners than I had seen in one place all summer. I went to the room, changed my shirt, rinsed out the old one in the sink and washed my face thoroughly. The water ran both hot and cold. I tested the hot water several times. *A novelty.* The toilet flushed. *Oh Joy.*

I walked through the town. It was more humid than Tansen. A water buffalo stood at a garbage pile next to a dog with no collar. The two animals munched on selected items as if they were tourists enjoying a buffet. I could see the ribs of the buffalo, the dog too for that matter. I walked further, to the landing dock past some Tibetans playing Sirangi, the little Nepali wooden fiddles they were trying to sell. They made it look easy to play. There was a small temple on an Island in the lake that might have been interesting. The weather was overcast and I decided not to go out on the water. The mountains would not be visible today. Turning back and walking south, I passed the former palace which now served as the military headquarters, complete with razor wire. Further along was a small Hindu shrine to Shiva which featured the statue of a cobra. Tibetan women were calling "Allemande?" so they could use their German skills to sell me jewelry from blankets laid out on the sidewalk. *Do I look German?*

It was the slow season and the shops were not crowded. There were no souvenir shops in Tansen and you could not buy any touristy items other than a few postcards. Here in Pokhara there was quite a selection including bookstores, T-shirts, and Tibetan items. There were also ATMs and western banks. Most of the books were about the Himalaya and trekking. I was looking for anything which related to the Magars but since the Magars are far from the Himalaya, I guess they were just not trendy enough, so I kept browsing. There were lots of books on Tibet. Pokhara has a sizeable Tibetan community, unlike Tansen. If there were Tibetans in Tansen, they blended in very well. I never saw even one Tibetan prayer flag in Tansen, ever. In the window of a bookstore at Lakeside, prominently on display, was a book devoted to the idea that Jesus Christ was actually a Hindu, and that He had spent his formative years in India studying Buddhism before returning to Nazareth to take up His ministry. *Wonder how that book would go over at the Guest House.*

Weeks earlier I had decided to accumulate the various items that a typical Magar Hill Woman would wear, and had gotten most of these in Tansen. I was still on the lookout for some shawls made of *pashmina*, the fine underbelly hair of a goat. *Pashmina* is the finest wool. With the nicest grade of *pashmina*, you could pull a full-sized shawl through a wedding ring, or so they said. Scarves made of *pashmina* are a trendy accessory in Paris and New York. Pokhara had a number of *pashmina* shops. I stopped at one place, prepared to receive the full sales pitch. The salesman was a young man with nice western-style clothes and oiled hair, who smiled broadly when I sat on one of the low wooden stools in the shop. His English was excellent, and he pulled out one shawl after another, until there were thirty or so shawls laid out before me. One at a time, I thought of the women in my life, conjuring up a mental picture of each and how they would act if they had one of these shawls. *Would they even know how to wear it?* The salesman quoted me a price in dollars, which was unusual for Nepal. He wanted dollars if at all possible. "I give you very good price."

I needed to convert the price back to Rupees to see for myself whether I was getting a bargain. I shook my head and told him no, I would not buy today after all, maybe tomorrow. Also, in Tansen the women favored one particular design style. I guess you would call it minimalist – just a few tasteful hand embroidered flowers or birds, with wide stitches. None of the embroidered shawls here had that kind of design. If I was going to get *pashmina* shawls, I wanted them to be similar to the ones I saw the local women wear every day. As I walked away I thought about shopping at Filene's Basement in Boston with my former wife – and I reassured myself that all the women in my life knew how to spot a bargain. They would not want me to spend more than I needed. I wondered whether they would enjoy the added element of negotiation to be found in Nepal.

Walking around Pokhara I saw a bar that advertised a nightly show with Nepal's only Pink Floyd cover band. The medical students had sucked down a few beers in this spot the previous week. I had no yearning to take in a Pink Floyd show today or any other day. A Korean restaurant and several Mexican places. I decided to eat at the hotel restaurant for dinner and take in the authentic folk dance show. It struck me that I was in my own self-contained little world. Compared to my working life at the hospital where I needed to talk all day long, this was relaxing – I did not have to talk to anybody. *It would have been great to share this with a woman,* I thought. *My daughters, or even my former wife or Celeste.* Most of the tourists seemed to be guys, like a group of thirty Boy Scouts from Belgium.

On the main street of Lakeside there was an internet café on the second floor above a restaurant and I climbed the circular metal staircase painted bright yellow. I could almost reach out and touch the electric wires jangling out of the transformer on the nearby pole. Somehow the wires here were all tangled, not neat the way an American linesman would have done, and I never figured out why they could not have done it more neatly. The internet was fast in Pokhara and the café here served pastries and coffee. I got an email from my former wife. She was concerned about my mental state. She asked if people in the local medical community at Tansen got Seasonal Affective Disorder during monsoon. My email reply was *Who needs Seasonal Affective Disorder when there are so many other bona fide reasons to be depressed?* I laughed to myself. *Too clever by half. But probably true.*

There was another email from Celeste. On June fourteenth, she went to Tara Puja, a type of Tibetan evening prayer which takes place on the full moon. Tara is the Goddess, and Celeste wished she had magical power. People there at the Tibetan temple in Honolulu had asked about me. She missed hearing me sing the way I did when I was happy, and life was boring. She hoped I was okay.

Back at the hotel, I fished through my daypack to find the book I had brought from the Guest House Library, *Annapurna* by Paul Herzog. Pokhara was mentioned prominently in the book, it was on the route that Herzog and his companions had taken to get to Annapurna. Herzog suffered severe frostbite when his gloves blew off during the descent of Annapurna, and in this very town, Herzog dictated his book while he recuperated from surgery to amputate his fingers and toes. *Now there was a guy who had been transformed when he came this way.* I read the book while sprawled lazily on the bed, enjoying the thick western-style mattress. I watched Bollywood MTV and caught the video from Kailash Kher titled *Saiyyan* which was a love song. Kailash used his soaring tenor to pour out his heart for a woman as he walked on the grounds of a palace in India. Most of his music is more electronic but in this video his voice shone with radiance. *That guy sure can sing.*

I put on my *topi* and the silk Hawaiian *aloha* shirt I had brought. They did not match, but the shirt was clean so I did not care. *None of the usual rules apply here anyway.* I chose a table where I could see the band. *Party of one.* The restaurant was mostly empty. Outside on the patio there were a dozen Japanese businessmen enjoying a barbecue under a blue tarp canopy. Six trekkers sprawled at a table by the wall, speaking German or Dutch. You could tell they were trekkers because of their clothes and the way they walked. Their faces were tan except for the area that showed a sunglass line, like raccoon eyes. The two women seemed to be saddle sore, and walked very stiffly.

Out of the corner of my eye I could see a person enter and sit down. A blond-haired woman. She was on the other side of a column. I held my glasses in my hand while I read the menu. She sat with her back to me and I couldn't make her out too clearly. I thought about saying something, and fidgeted in my seat as to how to approach this person. *Is she alone? The worst she can say is no.* So I got up and went over to speak to her.

"Excuse me; they say eating by yourself is bad for digestion. Why don't you come over and we can eat together?" She looked to be about thirty and I noticed what a thick single braid she had, long dirty-blond hair down her back. She wore a silver and turquoise ring on the middle finger of her right hand. She looked at me for a moment. She was trying to maintain eye contact but I distinctly thought she gave me the up-and-down glance. Then she smiled.

"I would love to have somebody to eat with. This is my only trip to Pokhara for this summer and I don't know anybody." She spoke in an Aussie accent, unmistakably broad. A bit grating, but measured and slow. *This was going to be interesting.* She had a nice smile and large brown eyes. She was pale with freckles.

"Well, my name is Joe. How do you do?" I mimicked my best British formality as she stood to shake hands, and I noticed that her hands were rough and fingernails broken. She had a strong grip for somebody so petite.

"Audrey, charmed." She made a slight curtsy. She looked over her shoulder at me as we walked back to my table. We sat across from each other. The Nepali band was starting to play on the other side of the patio. She wore a Magar-style red *cholo* blouse with a faded navy blue ankle length skirt and sandals. *Not a trekker.*

"What's up with the *cholo?*"

She smiled and sat a little straighter. "Do you like it?"

"I love the outfits but I didn't expect to see a western woman wearing a *cholo* when I came to Pokhara. Aren't you forgetting something?"

She looked down. "I don't think so..."

"Look again."

Another pause.

She held out her arms. "You mean bangles?"

"No. Aren't you supposed to be wearing a *patuka?*"

"You devil. And what, may I ask, are you doing with a *topi?*" *Feigned indignation.*

"I am using it to cover my head."

The waiter came around to take cocktail orders. Audrey asked for a Tuborg Beer and made a comment about how they could not have settled Australia without beer. *God, this is the same thing Barbara said.* I had not had a drink all summer, but ordered a Beefeater Gin and Tonic. *What the hell, I am on holiday.*

Audrey told me she wore the *cholo* because she was living with a Gurung family. She was an anthropology graduate student from Melbourne. And yes, she often wore a *patuka*.

"Where are you staying?" I asked.

"I'm observing the Gurungs in the area west of Annapurna. I have been living in a small village. It takes a full day just to walk to a paved road." This was her third trip to Nepal. The drinks came quickly and we made a toast to Pokhara and the Hotel Barahi. She emptied half the glass right there. *Pokhara was getting civilized just like Australia*, I thought. She ordered *shish kabob*, using rapid Nepali and joking with the waiter. I ordered Rogan Josh.

Despite the initial banter, Audrey carried herself in that self-contained way that I also noticed in the health workers from more rural areas of Nepal when they stayed at the Tansen Guest House. Or maybe it was a sense of focus – she projected a sense of calm. Or maybe it was just the same culture shock I was having myself.

"Field work – have you read *Love and Honor in the Himalayas?*" This was one of the books I read before going to Tansen where all the Magars were. It was easy to recall this book when she described her work.

"You know that book?" Audrey leaned forward in her chair.

"Of course I do. I love that book." *Love and Honor in the Himalayas* tells the story of village life in Nepal in a vernacular style, as if you were sitting in the living room of Ernestine McHugh, the author. The Gurungs are closely related to the Magars, which was why I bought it. The activity in the book took place less than fifty miles from Tansen.

"I love that book too. I am surprised to find somebody else who has read it."

By the time the second round of drinks arrived we agreed that the heart of the book was the scene where Ernestine's host family sister gets sick from typhoid and dies, while Ernestine lives. It is a beautifully written chapter, very moving and includes sections about the grief rituals of the village. Audrey sat in the chair but put her legs cross-legged in the lotus position and slowly undid her braid. She shook her hair loose. We had a third round. This time we toasted Ernestine McHugh.

She told me about her research focus. We also discussed Bollywood. She liked the same Kailash Kher video I had watched on the hotel cable channel.

So I managed to find the only other intellectual foreigner in Pokhara, I thought. She is single, unattached, and from a western country. And she has just come in from the countryside. I took a deep breath.

For her field work she visited nearby villages and did a lot of walking every day. She also was helping with the maize crop, which was why her hands were so rough. There was a pace to her field work, and she was enjoying just being part of the womenfolk. She was up early every morning to get water from the nearby stream that served as a tap in her village.

She asked what I was doing there.

"You are obviously not a trekker, mate."

"Was it the *topi* that gave it away? I am here from Tansen. I am not here to conquer the mountains. I am here to deal directly with the people of Nepal. I am working at a hospital for the summer."

"Are you...... a doctor?" she said as she touched her hand to her throat. *O God, I knew she would ask that*, I thought to myself.

"No, I am not. Everyone asks me that. I am a nurse and I teach nursing at the University." She brought her hand back down to her beer glass, holding it lightly and feeling the smoothness of the rim between her fingertips. She leaned back slightly.

"University? A faculty member? I say, how nice to meet a 'colleague.' I think we are the only two academics in Pokhara right now. Tell me more." She was obviously more relaxed and she was pretending at being more British, with a wry smile.

"A veritable cross-disciplinary colloquium if I do say so myself," I chimed in. *Two can put on airs. I was mimicking what I imagined Mark Powell might say.*

By this time the main course was set in front of us. I told her about Mission Hospital and the Pediatric Ward. I was making a conscious effort not to give too many graphic details of the burn victims. *That would probably just kill the conversation right there.* Instead I talked about offering hope to the mothers, and how I tended to identify with the children because I could think back to the time when my own kids were that age. I knew at the time it probably sounded like a play for sympathy, but hey, it was true. My voice cracked just a little and I stopped for a second. She put out her hand to touch mine and we made eye contact. *Maybe this is going to work after all.*

"I can tell you need to take your mind off work. You are a very caring man. Sounds like you really need this holiday." *I knew her tone of voice,* and I was a bit startled to hear it. It was low and a bit husky. I did not hear women speak to me in that tone very often these days – but I recognized the significance of it immediately. A few years back there had been a TV commercial for Cracklin Oat Bran in which a woman was at the breakfast table with a man asking, "Did you... take the last .... of the Cracklin Oat Bran?".... in the commercial it was a seductive voice, and what made the commercial so effective was the way it was used. *Who could resist such a tone of voice?* That tone from the commercial was the same sweet music my former wife would also use when whispering in my ear on the dance floor. *A siren call.* The last time I had heard it from my wife had been long before the divorce. *A tone of promise and intimacy.*

"Thank you. Sometimes I just need somebody to talk with and I could use a hug. I am around people all day but sometimes it's hard to relate. Don't you ever get lonely doing what you do?" *Two can use that tone.*

"Yes. My work is not near as difficult as yours, but I am the only one there who is not Nepali, sometimes it does get to me. I just need to come to a bigger town every now and then, speak English, and remember what it is like outside my village." We laughed about enjoying the hot showers, the flush toilets, the breakfast buffet, and fresh brewed coffee instead of instant. With a conspiratorial smile she leaned forward to tell me she shaved her legs the first day she arrived in Pokhara.

We finished our meal and I added mine to my hotel tab while she paid cash. There was an awkward moment as we stood up to walk out the door. She was ahead of me. She turned around. "It's a nice night for a little walkabout. I could use an escort to my hotel and I am not quite ready to turn in." *That crackling oat bran voice again.*

I opened the door for her and she looked up at me and winked as she walked through it. It was a bit misty and she waited outside the door. She was about six inches shorter than me, and I stepped a bit closer, searching for her hand. I ended up putting my arm around her waist instead as she rested hers on my shoulder.

The Nepali folk band played softly in the distance. She snuggled a little closer, so that our faces were about eight inches apart. I could feel her softness and warmth against my chest, and smell the perfume of her hair. It was nice. She closed her eyes and tilted her head up to me as she smiled.

The next morning I woke up feeling refreshed. We walked back to the Barahi. Breakfast was leisurely and we giggled as we sipped our coffee. "Aren't we a pair? You in that ridiculous *topi* and me in my *cholo*."

We said our goodbyes and Audrey left that day to return to the Gurung village while I went off to find the visa office. In the afternoon I napped. Dinner that night was alone, but I did not mind. The trip to Pokhara had been a success. I felt like a burden had been lifted from my shoulders. Saturday morning I took a taxi to the tourist bus depot. At first the plaza was full of western tourists, then their numbers diminished as they got sorted out and clambered onto chartered buses headed for various excursions. By the time my bus came there was one other westerner who climbed on with me. The Nepalis on board ignored us.

On the way back, there were no goats, no motion sickness and not a Maoist to be seen. I inspected my passport several times to look at the visa extension, which took up a whole page in the passport book. *Be Thou my Vision*, was going through my head, and I was trying to recall the words. I thought back to the other part of Matt's sermon, and steeling myself from sin.

To pass the time on the long bus ride, I tried to remember the Ten Commandments and I got the gist of them but could not put them in order. My little *Gideon's Bible* had only *the New Testament* not the *Old Testament*. I laughed when I had the thought: *According to this, I am going to hell when I die.*

In Search of Serenity

The bus from Pokhara did not go directly to Tansen. It left me off at Bartun, the name for a wide spot in the highway where the side road to Tansen veered off. The shuttle waited there for the Tansen passengers. It was like a jeep, with a canvas top, just slightly bigger, maybe the size of an SUV, carrying eighteen adults including the two-man crew, and eight children. Passengers hung on to the bumpers and running boards. As a westerner, I was grandly shown to a seat inside. *This was so-o-o-o typical of local conveyance.* The shuttle completed its trip to the Tansen bus plaza, and I walked the last mile, past the Hebron Church then up the hill overlooking the large valley. It was a sunny day. Below, the stream which meandered through the valley floor was now the color of *café au lait* due to the sediment-laden runoff. When I returned to the Guest House they told me that a rabid dog had bitten three people in Butwal. A team from Mission Hospital then dispensed rabies vaccine to a busload of people – thirty-five of them. Another man died of tetanus. Several people were admitted with snakebites, and fortunately all got the antivenin before being envenomated. An AIDS patient, another former sex slave, died of pneumonia. In other words, life had continued while I was gone. I met with Barbara to talk about maybe switching from Pediatrics to Adult Burns, but it turned out that there were only three adults in the Burn Unit and so no students were scheduled there. I was going to return to the exact place I had been. The glow from a successful trip to Pokhara lasted about as long as the bus ride home.

That evening I sat at the kitchen table in my small apartment in the Guest House, with my journal open in front of me to the next blank page. I held a four-color pen in my hand. There were ten of these pens tucked away with my luggage and I gave them to my new colleagues when I went to my first faculty meeting here at the Nursing School. With pen in hand I could think back to my normal life. Most of the baggage I brought with me to Tansen consisted of donated nursing textbooks. I was living out of one small suitcase for the whole three months. There were very few manifestations of my former life with me here.

Somehow that seemed so far away, as if Honolulu were the dream and this was the only reality. I gave up a lot of creature comforts to be here for the summer, and yet I did not actually miss Honolulu. I was settled into this particular life, and it was almost as if I had been doing this forever, and might still be doing it twenty years from now. The outside world no longer existed and the people at Mission Hospital were my only family, or so it seemed. Here in Tansen there was a very simple routine for everything, just as if I was in prison filling out a life sentence. Or perhaps I'd taken vows at a medieval monastery. Or lived on an island.

I wrote in the journal every day, starting with the date and a pair of numbers that kept track of how much time had elapsed and how much was left. This was 54/84 – the fifty-fourth day out of the eighty four days of the trip. A month to go and then the fall semester would start in Honolulu.

The whole episode with Dharsha and the mechanical ventilator now had an easy dreamlike quality to it. We made clinical decisions which were well thought out, but it was like working on a puzzle or playing Scrabble with friends. I had worked hard but in the back of my head I'd had a feeling all along that Dharsha would live.

And then the thought struck me about what Doctor Norma had said while Dharsha was still on the ventilator.

"God sent Joe Niemczura to us."

At the time I had not known what to say. A day or two later, when we thought that Dharsha was going to die despite our best efforts, I thought of the perfect rebuttal. If this was a world in which people are able to engage in immediate witty repartee I would have said to Norma, "That would only prove that God has a sense of humor."

I was searching for a way to express my thoughts for now. I had to set aside the ironic humor. I felt like crying when I thought of the health disaster that was Nepal. I found myself going back to the tune that was playing the day I first saw the burns on the legs of Kusmati, the Magar baby. It was *Tell Me Why*......

Ain't nothing but a heartache
Ain't nothing but a big mistake
I never want to hear you say
I want it that way.

I wondered if the Backstreet Boys had thought of the possible spiritual implications of their music. It was a song of sadness and questioning. Somehow this song put me in a mood to contemplate the hopelessness that some of patients were facing. *Go ahead. Ask. Ask God to' tell me why'...*

On Pediatrics the one unshakeable fact for me was that the element of enjoying the clinical decision-making as if it was a game, the element of fun and reward, was completely gone.

And I realized that *the point where the sense of adventure had disappeared was also the exact place where the actual Christian service began. Everything prior to that point was just lip service and going through the motions. The challenge was to find that place in myself where I could get over the shock of it. And do something about it.*

186

And actually serve.

If God sent me to Mission Hospital for any reason at all, maybe it was to be on the Pediatric Ward, doing what I am doing now.

Exactly what I am doing now. When this thought came, I needed to put the pen down. I put both hands on my face as I felt the flush of heat that came with the feeling of powerlessness. I prayed. It was a very simple prayer. *Please God. Help me get through this part.* I put the journal aside. One of the guys in the band had given me a small Gideon's New Testament English version. I opened it. *Start with Acts.* Acts of the Apostles was usually the first place the actual missionaries would turn. But in Acts, we are reading about people who already had faith – something which I was questioning – *where did faith come from?*

Certainly there was pain in the passion of Christ, but it was not Christ's pain that was speaking to me – it was my own, which was more akin to that of Christ's followers who watched the passion from a distance. *Tell me why* –

What was uppermost in my own mind was a feeling of questioning God, and being *witness* to suffering that now was uppermost in my mind. *Ain't nothing but a heartache* –

I thought of the resurrection and the Easter message – redemption and the end to eternal suffering. That was the message that propelled the Apostles and Saints, but somehow I did not think it would apply here, in the land of the Hindus. *Ain't nothing but a big mistake* –

The task of converting the Hindus to Christianity, something which the local Nepali Christians were trying to do, seemed overwhelming. I could not accept the idea that all these Hindu children would somehow be going to hell because of a loophole, or that their suffering was in any way due to the religion of their parents.

It occurred to me that Christ himself was serene for most of the actual passion. It was a question of anticipation.

What did He do in anticipation?

And that is how I got to the passage where Christ himself prayed for the strength to carry on. It is described in two passages; the first is *Luke*, Chapter 22, Verses 39 – 46. The second is *Mark*, Chapter 14, Verses 32-40. This scene is not described in *Matthew* or in *John*.

All that Jesus asked his disciples to do, in his own time of despair and grief, was to be at his side, stay awake, and pray. Christ Himself had prayed for greater faith and for the serenity to get through a difficult day. Here was the key to Christ's own suffering – the fact that He let go of His own sense of control and simply accepted what was to come. After that, the passion was an anticlimax.

God may have brought me to a hospital at the end of the earth, but God had not abandoned me here. I allowed myself to cry. Somehow this idea brought its own sense of serenity and relief for me. It was *okay* to have difficulty, it was *okay* to be bummed about the way things were, and it was *okay* to just take it one step at a time. It was *okay* to be there in Nepal and do what I could.

After that study, I brushed my teeth and went to bed. I prayed again, in the quiet darkness of rural Nepal. Outside it rained. I slept. I do not recall any dreams that night.

Will the Monsoon Ever Arrive?

The next day the alarm rang at five. I enjoyed my coffee and took the short walk to Pediatrics by six in the morning, my usual time. I hopped over the puddles in the stone pathway. The rhododendron at the junction was a burst of brilliant hues of lilac. I got to the eaves of the hospital and shook my umbrella as I collapsed it. I was now under the awnings of the hospital, sort of a galleria between buildings. The laundry staff was gathered for their morning meeting and I could see them through the laundry window as I walked past.

I suppose you are waiting for me to claim that somehow my religious insight had led me to acquire supernatural powers or that I could now somehow cure the kids so their burn injuries would improve overnight. No. I was the same guy with the same skill I had the day before. The only difference was that now I felt a lot more at peace with what I was trying to do there and that I was ready to give people the emotional support they needed as I worked to motivate and teach my batch of students.

God had not sent supernatural powers to me, but God had sent Mission Hospital. Despite the things they lacked here, what they did have was an astounding dedication and compassion. Maybe I was not going to get some kind of miracle, but wasn't it miracle enough that the Hospital was even here in the first place? Today, the dingy bricks seemed to take on a kind of strange beauty as I reflected on the effort it took to build this ramshackle collection of buildings, brick by brick, a bunch of small acts, taken in the aggregate, had produced an effect that exceeded the sum of the acts. When I got to the ward, I could look around the ward and remind myself that many of the patients were getting better. This had been true all along.

Around this time we had a twelve-year-old boy with meningitis. First they put him in one of the six-bed rooms. He had a rigid neck, fever, and was having seizures. His hands were cramped like a praying rabbit – an involuntary response known as decerebrate posturing. There had been other deaths from meningitis earlier in the summer. This boy was receiving chloramphenicol, our most potent antibiotic. The next day the boy had more seizures. The mom was in her late twenties.

At rounds Norma turned to me and said in English, "The plain truth is, they brought this kid in too late and I think he is going to die. I am not planning to lay a guilt trip on the mom for this, but it is tragic." She and I both looked at the mom, who did not speak English. The mom was trying to read our expressions, sitting quietly and waiting for an explanation in Nepali. Norma could speak Nepali but for something sensitive like this, used the nurse to translate. She listed the things we were doing to save the boy. "I will have the hospital Chaplain stop by and talk with this family. That's about all that is left."

Later that morning, the nurses moved the boy to a private room near the nurse's station. This room was often used for such cases. It was a place where he could die in peace, and the family could be with him and not have an audience of strangers. We could avoid a scene that would upset the rest of the patients and their families. He could just quietly float away from shore. Until.

The next day the door to his room was shut as I went by on the way to rounds. *Not a good sign.* I was expecting the room to be empty. But we made our way down the list and the news was good. He was sleeping in a relaxed position on his side. No fever. He had not had further seizures. He had taken some water by mouth and eaten a bit. Mom was more relaxed.

Norma was happy, "Sometimes they just turn the corner. I really thought he was done. A bit of prayer is always good." A few days later he was discharged.

The students made a checklist of the day's dressing changes, mostly the same patients, and I could feel that I was more relaxed, not so battered by the sights and sounds. I found that I was not so abrupt with the students as I had been, and a few times I actually smiled. Also, they seemed to be grasping the way I wanted them to perform, and learning to anticipate the things I had been trying to get them to do that would make it go easier. It all flowed and I wished I had felt this sense of flow before; but then it occurred to me that anybody who wanted to get to this place had to do a lot of psychological work to prepare for the level at which events would unfold naturally and the team would work like a well-oiled machine.

One day I had to go home for lunch because Bimla had made *samosas* that were getting stale and I wanted to eat them before she returned the next day to cook more. There were a dozen sugar cookies in the bowl, and little black ants crawled on them. I brushed the ants off and reconstituted some powered milk with cold water. I dipped the cookies in the milk and thought of my parents in Honolulu and the cookie jar we had when I was a kid and which was now in the possession of my daughter. I stuffed the rest of the cookies in my pocket and headed back to work. On the way there I saw one of the American medical students so I pulled a cookie out of my pocket and offered it to him.

"Wait, did you just pull that out of your pocket?"

"Yes."

"Well, was it in a bag?"

"No."

"Hey, I don't want it, it's covered in dirt."

"You are kidding, right? I am offering you a cookie and you are worried about a little dirt? What, germs? Do you have any idea as to how many germs you are exposed to just by walking into the hospital? You may already sero-converted to TB and you don't know it. Have you thought about that? And you are worried about a sugar cookie?"

"I don't know, man— "

Just then Samuel came hurrying on by. I knew what a busy schedule he had, maybe he had skipped lunch. I said, "Hey Samuel, your mother called."

He stopped and grinned "Oh, what did she say?"

"She said you have been a very good boy and she wants you to have these." I pulled three cookies out of my pocket and held them out. He smiled, took them and bit into one, putting the others in his pocket.

"Thanks! These hit the spot. Gotta go!" and he was off.

The American student said, "Well they can't be that bad —" and he took two. He smiled when he bit into the first one.

When I was relaxed I was better able to relate to the kids. Ramesh was the boy with TB of the shin bone. All day he sat in bed, waiting to get better, which was taking time. His grandfather sometimes sat with him. We never saw his parents and the rumor was that they were dead. Nobody knew for sure. Ramesh needed to play but was hampered by his need for a walker. One day I playfully gave Ramesh my torch. He would hold it for an hour in the morning and shine it on passersby. I taught him how to make the hand gestures that went with *Junior Birdman*. He would do it whenever he saw me. It was a game. I would sometimes put my *topi* on his head.

The medical side of the ward was where the children with pneumonia were housed. I brought my camera one day and was taking pictures of the patients and their mothers. I noticed one baby's mom who could not have been more than twenty-five years old. As she held the baby, I noticed that she had fingernail clubbing and a slight barrel chest, both of which are signs of chronic lung disease. The usual kitchen in Nepal is an open-topped clay wood stove with no chimney. This woman probably stayed near a smoky fire every day, all day. *No wonder the child had pneumonia.* I wondered what mom's lungs would be like in another five years.

Another child with pneumonia was thin as a rail, with a big belly, thin hair, arms and legs like sticks with huge knees. I thought maybe he also had a "rachitic rosary," a sign of rickets, but Norma didn't think it was quite that bad. *This child is a victim of plain old starvation.* Almost fifty percent of children in Nepal are so far behind on the growth chart that their growth will be stunted for life. On discharge, he was sent to our Nutritional Resource Center to gain weight.

The chartered bus to Pokhara departed with its load of *videshis* taking their holiday. That same day the rains finally, truly, irrevocably came. The monsoon had truly begun, more than month late. For the first two days it rained continuously. At the hospital the rain drummed on the tin roof and we all needed to stand closer to hear one another. Then it would have periods of slower and faster rain but it never really stopped for fifteen days, the rest of the time I was there. The fine red dust that covered everything was replaced by tracked-in mud. The daily temperature dropped twenty degrees, and it was now only about eighty degrees during the daytime, which seemed cold to many of the locals.

The roads became muddy. My favorite walking route between the hospital and the *Bajar* was studded with small landslides, each about the size of a dump truck load of dirt. There were reports of larger landslides and rockslides on the mountain road to Tansen from the Terai, and that week the Buck was delayed for hours, arriving well after dark. In the morning, the waiting room at the hospital was only half full, and the crowd that had formerly gathered at the water tap by the ER was smaller since everyone could collect rainwater from their own roof.

Monsoon is celebrated in the music and literature of South Asia as a time of release from the usual constraints of society. A time of sensuality. Or so they say. The only difference I noticed was that the women would all wear their saris a little higher out of the mud, and some ankle would be showing. O My God! The women of Nepal are extremely modest and you normally never see even the least little bit of a woman's body below the waist. When the Nepalis would see a western woman in a short skirt, this unwritten rule leads them to conclude that western women were all harlots. In Tansen the female missionaries were careful to observe local customs for that reason. But now, to keep the hem of their *saris* clean, the local women were forced to hold up the cloth and display themselves. *Ankles on display!* Men would also roll up their trouser legs while walking outdoors. At the *Bajar*, it was not unusual to see two men, or two women, walking arm in arm to share the same umbrella.

Over the next few days after the beginning of monsoon, children were discharged but fewer were admitted. The census in Pediatrics dropped to about thirty – half of what it had been. Movement had become hampered and people could not make their way to the hospital. The weather in Nepal had shut the place down just as if it had been a blizzard in New England.

The Missionary Position and Others

In the Guidebook section on Tansen, there was reference to the erotic carvings on the struts of the local Newari temple. Earlier that summer during the pre-monsoon I took a trip to see the carvings. There they were, in cracked wood, stained by pigeon droppings. The first one was the missionary position. *Of course.* I stepped up to get a closer look, but I looked around and soon reconsidered. During the hot dusty pre-monsoon there was always a crowd of bathers at the nearby tap, so I did not wish to look like I was a voyeur, and risk offending the women's sense of propriety. I was always worried somebody would come after me with a bamboo *lathi* and I would get thrashed. Now that the monsoon was here, everyone could collect all the water they needed right at their house, just by setting out a row of pots under the drip line. I walked to the temple neighborhood. Not far away, water rushed down Steep Street in a torrent. Nobody was at the tap. I took my camera out of the waterproof case and snapped away, one shot each for the sixteen struts. The photos came out very clear.

The next day the *videshis* were conducting a tag sale to raise money for the mission school and I pulled out my camera which had the pictures on the viewer. A small knot of people gathered. The medical students were snickering as they joked about which positions they had tried and which were their favorites. Tom and Karen Rockland came over. When they saw the knot of people they wanted to see what was going on.

Karen Rockland was the Canadian teacher at the one-room school house. Karen was blond and attractive, with the sort of bubbly outgoing positivism you would expect from an elementary school teacher. Tom was going bald though he was only thirty, and every day he trooped down to the hospital pharmacy where he worked with the Nepali staff.

"I know it's not glamorous but I am here to serve, any way I can, and this is what I do," he said to me.

They were a pleasant couple, and Karen's job as a teacher was critical to the success of the Missionary community. The kids and the parents loved her and I could see why. But I did not interact with them much because I had no children at the school.

So when Tom and Karen wanted to see the photos I said, "You may not be old enough to see these." But Tom and Karen persisted so I showed them one which depicted three very supple people, and their mouths dropped.

She asked, "Are those carvings here? In *this* town?"

Karen could recite much of the *Bible* from memory, but it was then I realized that she probably had not studied anything about Hinduism or Buddhism, and most certainly had not looked at the *Kama Sutra*. She had never been to the foot of Steep Street in the *Bajar* where the temple was located, even after a year of mission work here. She mainly walked between her apartment and the school and stayed on the grounds behind the wall.

Later that week I was invited to the Rockland's for dinner. They were planning to take two weeks in Hawaii at Christmas for a vacation after two years in Nepal, and they wanted advice regarding things to see and do at Waikiki.

Stepping into the Rockland's apartment, I crossed a magical invisible boundary, as if I had been transported to rural Ontario. There was nothing inside to remind the occupants that we were in South Asia. Hockey magnets held the latest school work to the metal door of the fridge. Near the TV were all the latest DVDs for the kids. Posters of the Canadian Rockies were tacked to the wall. The carpet was strewn with the usual American toys. Karen showed me the contents of the fridge. She was proud to have western food and canned goods, and told me of the ingenuity in obtaining the brands with which she was familiar, especially the cheese.

Dinner was tuna noodle casserole, with a special dessert – apple pie. We said grace at the dinner table. The whole effect reminded me of growing up the fifties. Wholesome. I suppose that if I were to live in Ontario in the wintertime, this was exactly how I would spend an evening at home while the wind howled outside. On a long winter night we would be settling in to await the coming of Spring. *But there was no weather from which to be insulated. It was Nepal out there.*

At dinner the four-year-old daughter asked, "Why do you have such a fat belly?" Tom and Karen paused, horrified that the decorum had been broken.

With a straight face I solemnly answered, "Because I used to like to drink beer. If you drink beer you get fat."

That relieved the tension and we changed the topic. Karen passed the green beans. After dinner, we all talked about the beaches and activities for tourists in Hawaii. The family listened eagerly while Tom took notes on his laptop. Somehow the erotic struts on the temple never came up during the conversation.

Later, before the kids went to bed, I got to hold the Gerbils. It was a fine evening.

Sanjita Takes a Vacation

One day in late July, Sanjita took me aside just after report and told me, "There is something important we need to talk about, I have a favor to ask of you." I was a bit surprised, because she used *that* voice... *the crackling oat bran voice.*

This must be important, I thought. *I have never once heard Sanjita use that tone, not with me or with anyone.* I thought of the last woman who had used that tone of voice with me, and the thought put me in a good mood. So I smiled. What she wanted was to take a quick, four-day vacation to visit her family. Would I mind covering the students on Pediatrics by myself?

Sanjita was from a city in the *Terai* where her mother and sisters still lived. Her father was an agricultural outreach specialist for the Nepali government. He specialized in rice growing, and she once told me that when she was a little girl she remembered when small groups of local farmers would come to the door of her house in the evenings, bringing rice plants, roots and all. Her father would beckon them to sit in a circle on the floor while he examined the plants by lamplight, a healer of plants giving a prognosis. She recalled seeing their dark faces and white turbans shine in the flickering lamplight. She looked at me proudly as she described this. Now, to comply with a government policy, her father was transferred to a posting to Nepalganj in western Nepal for a year, an involuntary exile from Sanjita's mother, a schoolteacher. He would be coming home for a week. Sanjita wanted to join her brother and sister as they greeted their dad for the first time in six months.

I had to say yes. I told her I knew what it was like to miss your parents, and she would owe me one. She was very happy and a look of outright joy came over her face. She jumped up and down like a seven-year-old. She left later that same day for home.

The census was forty-four, with six empty beds and nobody on pallets. The next four days were busy for me, as I was now involved in the full range of activities of clinical supervision – morning observation of students doing histories and physicals, then dressings, then looking at new orders, then supervising students as they gave medications to the children.

In one bed was a child who had been attacked by a wild monkey. This was the first time I had seen monkey bites. The girl was six years old, had been playing in the school yard after her friends left. It was just one monkey. I suppose I was expecting to find actual bite marks, like two parentheses ( ), but that is not how monkeys attack. They have sharp incisors, and the wounds on the child's arms and legs were long and deep as if she had been sliced multiple times with a steak knife. Her legs were swollen, and the surgeons asked us to remove every other suture, alternating, to allow the edema fluid to drain out. She got a tetanus shot and rabies prophylaxis and was given antibiotics. She ultimately did okay and was discharged. This was one more hazard of rural Nepal. Later when I was in Kathmandu I was careful around the semi-wild monkeys of Pashupattinath and Sangkhu. *Never make eye contact with a wild monkey. It is considered to be "threat behavior."*

Another six-year-old was admitted for reconstructive surgery on his left arm. This child had broken his forearm just above the wrist the previous year. He broke both bones, the radius and the ulna, in what is called a "Colle's fracture." These happen all the time, especially with a rambunctious kid like this guy. It is an easy fracture to fix. It could have been repaired in ten minutes without making an incision. Just a little anesthesia, set it into place, another X-Ray, and put on a plaster cast. But this child's parents never brought him to the hospital. Now he had a forearm that made a zigzag. He could use his fingers but the hand was weak. In a normal hand the tendons function like pulleys but this boy's hand functioned as if they were all off the track where his wrist had healed improperly. He was going to need a series of surgeries if he was to ever use that hand with any kind of strength. He was a rambunctious child and the cast on his arm did not prevent him from running around the ward getting into trouble. One morning he used his good hand to make a gesture at me which stopped me dead in my tracks – he had just given me *the finger!* I asked one of the students what the gesture meant when used in Nepal, and it means, *We are number one.* I did not have my camera with me, but brought it from my apartment later that day, and took a photo. Of all the pictures I brought back, that one gets more comments than any other. *I did not teach him that gesture. I swear.*

At ten in the morning while the patients ate their *dal-bhaat*, Rati came down from Maternity to check on me. She smiled a lot. When she spoke she seemed to be cooing like a dove. In the canteen one day I learned through the grapevine that one of the interns had told her my secret – that I was actually single, not married as I had been telling people. I thought Rati was more friendly than usual. I noticed that she stood just a bit closer than formerly, and acted a bit more coy, with her eyes just a bit downcast. *She really was attractive.* Rati smelled nice. *Was that perfume?* I knew I would be leaving in ten more days. I made a conscious effort to just enjoy being in her presence, and simply take deep breaths, Smiling as I noticed the freckles on the back of her neck. *Things were okay on Pediatrics. Really.* There were long pauses in the conversation.

Rati was tall and willowy, and as she walked away I had this idea that she was accentuating the way her frame curved as she walked. She looked over her shoulder and smiled as she went around the corner on the way back to the Maternity Ward.

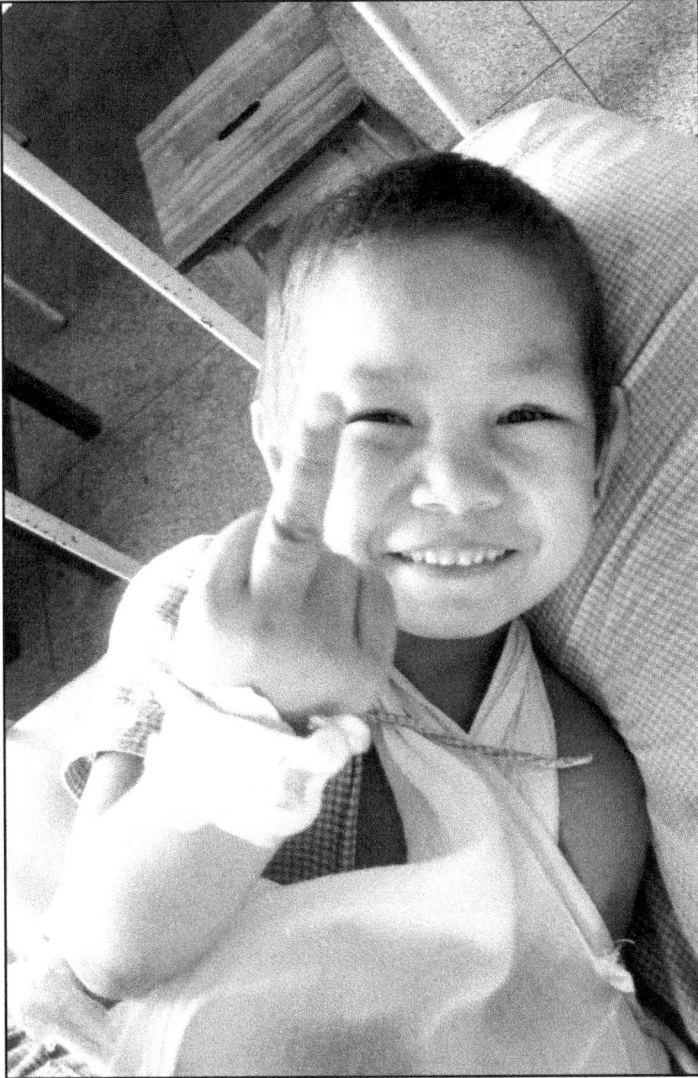

This gesture has a different meaning in Nepali than it does in English. This boy was rambunctious and exuberantly full of life between surgeries on his wrist.

Padma Visits Pediatrics

With only a week to go, Al and Padma were itching to move on to their next adventure. Al was saying how he seemed to be a really shy guy around women, and he was grateful that Miss Boston would even give him a second look. So we teased Al and the other medical student from Seattle about dumping their present girlfriends now that they had some mojo after spending the summer in Tansen. Al retorted by saying to me at least he *had* a girlfriend. He seemed to catch himself and apologized if he had struck too close to home. I looked at him. I thought of what to say about my friend from Melbourne, and decided to say nothing.

In Afghanistan, the Taliban had kidnapped two dozen Christian workers from a South Korean relief organization. Over the next several days, there was worldwide media coverage to cover the unfolding events. The Taliban murdered several of the missionaries in cold blood to heighten the pressure on the South Korean government. The rest remained hostages. There was a tangible sense of solidarity among the *videshis* in Tansen, and the progress of negotiations was reported along the grapevine each day. Every one in Tansen prayed for the Korean missionaries. With a shock, we wondered if Park was among the captives. *What a twist of fate.* Later somebody told us that Park was still in Seoul and never went to Afghanistan. This was the first time we talked about Park since he left. We were all relieved when the Korean hostages were released.

Talk at the dinner table then turned to the subject of dealing with the stress on Pediatrics. Al and I were talking about how rough Pediatrics had been, and speculating about how the long term doctors dealt with the stress. Samuel had confided in Al that he too cried some days. *Even Samuel, who was a rock of faith.* I was not the only one. We were trying to think of a Pediatric Ward in the US or UK that got cases like the ones here. Tansen, we agreed, had a Pediatrics department that was unlike anywhere else in our experience. Amidst this discussion, Padma had been silent but interjected, "Surely it can't be all that bad."

I turned to her and said, "What do you know about it? You have been enjoying yourself way too much up there in the Maternity building. Things are happy up there. You have been insulated from what has been happening here. In your own little bubble. You need to just spend one day on the Surgical side of Pediatrics with me and observe some dressing changes."

That night I had a dream about wounds. In my dream, I had a deep wound on my own leg behind the knee. Strangely, I could lift it over my shoulder to get an effortless look at it. I am not that flexible in real life. Al was shining the torch on it while I calmly probed, looking for the nerves, tendons, and arteries. I checked the margins of the wound for tunneling. In the dream it did not hurt. In the dream I remember thinking *I wonder when it will be ready for grafting?*

The next day Padma came to Pediatrics in the morning. She was on her way to the Outpatient Postpartum Clinic. I arranged to get her when it was time for the dressing on our two small burn victims. She came by just as we were removing the old dressing from Kusmati. Padma brought her camera and did what I could never do – took a photo of the wounds. She started out with her normal sunny disposition, but became thoughtful as she watched. The next patient was Akash. She took a picture of Akash with the dressing still on, and my own hand in the photo. There are very few other pictures in my collection in which I appear. I took a thousand photos over the summer but never appeared in them myself.

That evening was the beginning of the new month, the month of "*mehandi lagaunu.*" In late July, a new season begins in the Hindu worship calendar. Padma did not join us for dinner. Instead, she went to a small gathering of women at the home of one of the maternity nurses, ate there, and joined the others as they decorated their hands with *mehandhi.* The designs were fanciful and hers included an owl on the palm. *Mehandhi* is said to ward off snakes and scorpions. It is a vegetable dye also known as henna. Once applied it may not wear off for weeks. She showed off her new art work when she got in.

The next Monday one of the unmarried nurses was preparing the meds in the Pediatric nurse's station and just dropped to the floor. The other nurses matter-of-factly revived her, giving her some juice and holding her legs up so the blood would rush to her head. Until she got on her feet again, there was a momentary stir on the ward, with a crowd of nurses and other patients standing around her in a circle. One of the other nurses took over the meds. Later, when she returned, I asked her how she was feeling and she told me that during this month, the custom is to fast every Monday. She said while fasting, every unmarried woman is supposed to wear red, and pray that her future husband will be handsome and kind. The women also switch from red bangles to green. I made a note to myself to see whether Rati was wearing bangles and what color they might be.

The last night before Padma left, to be followed by Al two days later, Ellie and I joined them for a farewell dinner. We were joined by a couple of the new medical students who would be staying through the fall. We thought of going to Nanglo's, but settled on a different place – one which was rumored to have the best *momo* in Tansen. Up the hill from Nanglo's and around the corner there was this hole-in-the-wall joint which had been a private residence. This was located in downtown Tansen on a side street just off the main *Bajar*. You would order a plate or two of *momo* at a time, dip them in *achaar*, and wash them down with beer.

The ceiling was low, which forced us to bow our head, and the lintels over the doors were even lower. Each whitewashed room was furnished with a simple table with benches on either side. We ate plates of *momo* with *achaar*, and I sipped a lemon soda. Al talked about Tibet and his much-anticipated rendezvous with *The Fabulous Miss Boston*. I had been waiting for just the right moment to share some practical entomology that I had come across, and now was the time to share it with the group. While looking through a shelf in the Pediatric Ward, I had come across a dusty book from 1959 titled *Aids to Tropical Nursing*, and in it there was an old-timey illustration that depicted the differences between various species of mosquitoes in ways you could see with the naked eye. I found it fascinating. This is important in case you are in a malaria area. The anopheles mosquito is to be avoided.

I started to share this with the group. "You could tell if it was an anopheles by examining the angle of its hind end while the mosquito inserted its proboscis into your skin." At this, I was interrupted by a chorus of jeers and laughter, and several of them drummed their fists on the table.

"Joe! If you are in a malaria area, and mosquitoes land on you, KILL THEM ALL! You are MISSING the POINT!" Somehow this had escaped me, but once they said it, the logic was so obvious that I joined them in laughing at myself.

After we shared about ten plates of *momo* and several rounds of beer, I opened the small bag that had been under the table 'til now. First I gave Al a small book on Buddhism I found in a bookstore in Pokhara. Then, on behalf of all the guys at the Guest House, I gave Padma a *cholo* of her very own. Earlier in the summer I had taken note of Padma's size. Padma was delighted to see a *cholo* that had been made just for her, using a nice grade of *Palpali Dhaka* cloth and lined in red. She stood up and tried it on. She was the center of attention, and other customers crowded around to get a look as she tied the ties. The *cholo* fit like a glove. She started to sit down but I said, "wait!" Then I pulled out a five-meter-long *patuka* in bright yellow. Al lurched to a standing position, and held one end to Padma's bellybutton as I got up and stretched it out, stooping my head to walk into the other small room of the restaurant with the other end of the fabric. Padma held her arms up like a ballet dancer and twirled to reel it in. The onlookers gave a drunken cheer with a few whoops mixed in, and one of the American med students howled like a coyote. She kept it on for the rest of the evening, wearing it as we walked back to the Guest House. To get there we had to go through the hospital, and the *Chowkidar* smiled broadly as he let us in through the gate to the ER on our way.

Padma got on the Buck the next day at six in the morning. I thought of going down to see her off but it was raining so I slept late instead. Like so many other UMN people in transit, she would stay at the Salome Guest House in Patan. She was not sure how long she would be in Kathmandu, since she needed to go to the Indian embassy and apply in person for a visa for India, which sometimes took a few days. I was not sure I would see her again. Al rode to Kathmandu a few days later with a doctor who was driving that way.

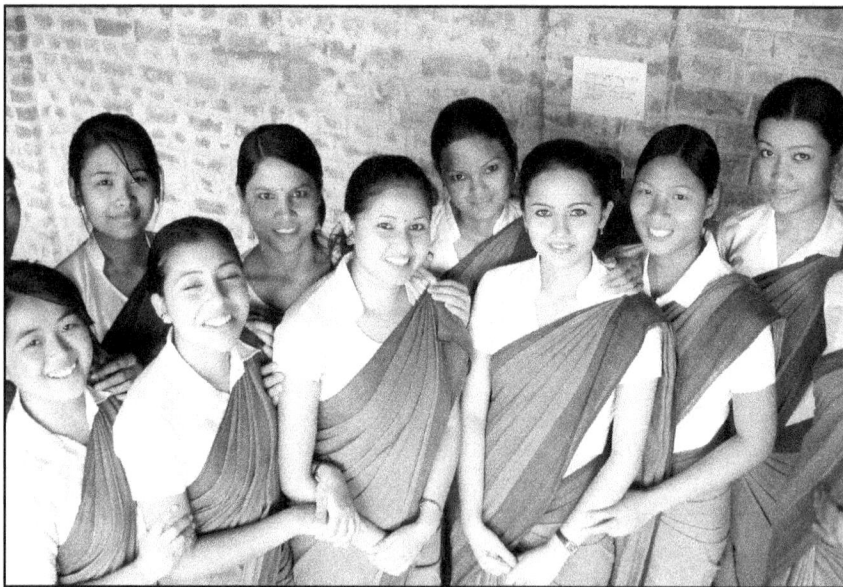

TNS students in the uniform they wear on class day. Purple and white. Students were not allowed to appear in public unless they wore either the work uniform or the class sari.

Saying Goodbye to the Students

The last two weeks before Al and Padma left were ones in which I was in the rhythm of the work. Each day I listened to report on the ward, then excused myself to attend Morning Prayer with the medical staff, and returned to Pediatrics to work with Sanjita and the students. One day, Surendra was holding a paper bag as he entered the conference room where the meeting was held. When the time came to report on the number of admissions, he stood up to announce that two more people were admitted with snakebite. These victims managed to capture their assailant and bring it to the hospital with them, alive and unharmed. Surendra then unveiled a peanut-butter jar with a bright green snake inside. It was a tree viper. The venom causes coagulopathy, and there is no antivenin for this particular snake, the victim is observed for blood clotting problems instead.

"Where are the people from?" Ellie asked.

"They live in the *Gairegau* neighborhood about a half-mile from here." This brought titters of nervous laugher. We all knew that *Gairegau* was where Ellie and Will and all the senior *videshi* medical personnel lived with their families. Ellie looked around and saw the opportunity; he took a moment to decide how to respond.

"I believe it is against Mission Hospital policy for snakes to inhabit that neighborhood." This was delivered in a deadpan tone, to twitters of laughter. He sat down.

For the next three days, the tree viper was alive in the Peanut Butter jar on the shelf next to the other samples. I borrowed it to show every one on Pediatrics. I showed it to Sanjita who jumped just as if she was a school girl. Then Surendra sent it to snake heaven. It will stay on the ER shelf until it loses its color and another one is brought in.

We arranged for a Wednesday toot on mechanical ventilation for the nursing staff which served to reinforce the experience with Dharsha. Shushila, the head nurse from Medical, served as my translator, and I felt good that the nurses would be able to do this skill without me if they needed it again. Seventy nurses and students came to the toot, the best attendance they ever had. I was humbled by this. Overall, I was at peace, and the sense of turmoil had dimmed. We changed Kusmati's leg dressings as well as Akash's head wound just about every day.

July twenty-seventh came, and this was to be the last day on Pediatrics for this group of students. They would be moving on to Maternity. A new batch would start Monday. At noon we were done with the dressing changes. I summoned the group together in the corridor outside the nurse's station. For the last time I held out my right hand at waist level, the signal to stand close for a small conference. They looked at each other and giggled a bit as usual while they made the same gesture, like a high school sports team. They stood a little closer, some of the girls putting their other arm around the waist of the girl ahead of them. They enjoyed being able to do a group cuddle like this.

I said, "This is the last time we will be together because I leave next week. I know that I was tough with you at times but I want you all to know that I appreciated the hard work you did. I apologize for the times I was angry with you." I looked around from face to face. This group of seventeen-year-old girls had been through a lot with me, with the high census and the dressing changes and the medications and – everything – learning about compartment syndrome, neuro checks, sternal retractions, stranger anxiety, omphocele, breastfeeding support, dying children, ostomy and diabetic teaching, monkey bites and enemas to kids with worm impactions. It occurred to me that they had proven themselves. They had grown.

Then Karuna, the informal leader of the group, took a deep breath and spoke up. "Joe Sar, you were tough and demanding but we all want to thank you. We knew that you were sharing things we would need. Most of all, we want you to know that you taught us all, the way a nurse should be. We could see that you loved these children and you taught all of us how to love these children. We will never forget the way you taught us."

There was a quiet *thank you*, and as I shook hands with each of them, I made eye contact and told them that I thought they would be wonderful nurses someday. As I walked out I found myself repeating what she said, turning it over in my mind. *All the work was worthwhile. All the effort had brought something here.* And I left for the day.

The next day was Saturday. I brought my trumpet to the Nepali Church for the last time, and played with the band. It was rainy. The pastor started the sermon by comparing the passages in the *Old Testament* in which various prophets went head-to-head with pagan priests to call down fire or produce miracles. These were colorful tales of earthquakes, snakes, lightning bolts, locusts, plagues and time standing still. He told the congregation to stay away from the temptation to decide for God on the basis of supernatural abilities. "Focus on the lived experience of Jesus Christ, the person who walked the earth, and follow His example."

On the way back, I decided to cut through the Pediatric Ward on my way to the apartment. As I walked down the hall, I passed the door to the treatment room, which was shut. Through it, I could hear a characteristic high-pitched cry of a child in pain. *I know who that is. I* stopped for a moment, then kept walking. I said a prayer as I went. *God bless every child, every mother, here.*

The new group of students started the following Monday, but I stayed home and packed my belongings. In the afternoon there was a tea at the Nursing School. The other faculty members presented me with a necktie made of *Palpali Dhaka*. I never wear neckties in Honolulu. I accepted it graciously. We all said nice things. The census on Pediatrics was still low. Sanjita would do just fine.

Leaving Tansen

It would take ten hours of travel on the roads to get from Tansen to Kathmandu. I wanted to leave plenty of travel time before my flight out so that if a *bandh* or a rockslide were to block the way, I would still get to the airport on time. So I planned to leave Tansen August 1ˢᵗ on the Buck. That gave me eight days of tourist-like sightseeing before departure.

The day after my arrival had been my only full day in the Kathmandu Valley and I recalled the sensory overload as I explored Patan Durbar Square on foot, walking through the crowded marketplace and having the sensation of being the only Caucasian in a crowd of thousands. The crowded vitality of Patan had been imprinted on my mind. Throughout the whole summer I had been thinking I would not be able to navigate the entire city myself. My plan would be to give myself a few days after leaving Tansen, but mainly do more mellow sightseeing elsewhere. And so, I had hardly even read the sections in my Guidebook that dealt with Kathmandu or the Kathmandu Valley.

My daydream was to spend a week in Chitwan National Park, located in the *Terai*, where a large swath of the jungle, wetlands and forest was still intact. Chitwan is famous for bird watching and wildlife viewing. At times in the evening in Tansen I would read the Chitwan section of the guidebook and daydream about walking in the forest, looking for birds with a guide. I am not much of a "birder," but I brought my binoculars with me as well as a copy of the book, *Birds of Nepal*. My older brother works in Houston and prides himself on his knowledge of the birds of Texas. When I planned the trip I invited him to visit Nepal with me but he was unable to get time off, and I teased him saying that I would go bird watching on his behalf so that he could enjoy Nepal vicariously. In Tansen I could hear the calls of many species but the thick vegetation of the broadleaf forest made it difficult to get a visual sighting. I was too busy with clinical work to spend as much time birding as I wished while I was there.

And now that I had the time to spend, the monsoon was not cooperating. Whole villages in the *Terai*, where Chitwan is located, were being flooded. I was getting lots of advice not to go there. The Buck always brought a copy of the *Kathmandu Post* to put in the sitting room of the Guest House. The *Kathmandu Post* ran a sensationalist headline on the front page about the number of deaths in the *Terai* due to the flood. Ellie and others told me not to go. "Of course, the elephant ride would have been great. When I took my family to Chitwan, we took the elephant ride. We had to go down a steep embankment and the highlight of the trip was when the elephant slid down the bank on her arse. With us on board!"

Thinking back to when I first arrived, I reflected on my own readiness for Kathmandu. The first day in Nepal was a huge sensory overload, magnified by fear of the unknown. That was nine weeks ago, and I was now wise to the ways of Nepal so as I read the guidebook, I found myself getting excited about the trip to Kathmandu.

Further back, in the same issue of the *Kathmandu Post,* I found an encouraging article. There are seven World Heritage Sites in the Kathmandu Valley as listed by UNESCO. They are Pashupattinath, Boudhanath, Swayambunath, Kathmandu Durbar Square, Patan Durbar Square, Changu Narayan, and Bhaktapur. Mysterious and magical names. To these, the guidebook added Ason Tole, a neighborhood downtown.

Now that I had been out of the bubble, I would not be satisfied unless I could get a feel for the way that people lived in the Kathmandu Valley, the way they conducted their daily lives. I did not want to feel hurried as I visited these places. Pashupattinath for example, is a holy site for Hindu cremations and after all that happened in Tansen, I felt it would be disrespectful to feel pressured by time the day that I visited Pashupattinath. I was not sure I was ready for Pashupattinath. My plan was to budget enough time to spend a full day at each of the seven sites on the list, and to be open to other things that came up.

The Buck did not bring me directly to the Guest House this time. No more coddling. Got off, thanked the crew, *Namaste,* and loaded my baggage into a taxi. I still remembered how to get to the Salome Guest House. It was the same Guest House I stayed at when I arrived, run by Christian Nepalis.

The Salome Guest House seemed like home now. The *didi* answered the door and smiled when she saw me. I knew how the bathroom worked and where to put my groceries. Best of all, Padma was there in a nearby room. She spent a week in Kathmandu while her visa request to India was processed, but today she got word that the visa to India was approved. She picked up her passport and she would leave in the morning. In Tansen, Padma and I had not said a proper good bye with a hug. Now she came out to greet me with one.

Padma filled me in on her time in the Valley. She cried when she first arrived in Kathmandu. She was feeling the same separation and loss from the Tansen community that I was feeling. *Like leaving a cult,* I thought. She made her way to the Indian embassy the first day, then one by one to the places I was planning to go. Seeing her made me feel as though I was with a member of my own family or somebody whom I had known forever.

She had not seen Al since she arrived. First he was bungee jumping and then river rafting. Al had only just returned to Kathmandu for a bit before he would take Miss Boston to Tibet. I took a shower and we got a taxi to Thamel, the district where all the tourist hotels and bars are located. We headed off to Fire & Ice, a restaurant located on the edge of the Thamel district.

Looking out the window of the taxi this time, Kathmandu no longer seemed as intimidating as I recalled from my arrival. The crowds? Familiar. The vehicles, the cows, the noise, everything – was somehow okay. I had learned a lot about Nepal and I was now ready to enjoy this city. The sights were the same; it was me that had changed.

The taxi stopped outside Fire and Ice. Through the plate glass we could see hanging ferns, abstract art with indirect lighting, and well-dressed patrons in padded chairs lingering over drinks.

"Al says it's the best pizza place in Kathmandu," said Padma, and I could see why. The atmosphere was just what you would get in any city in the US. Inside, the air conditioning was noticeable and my glasses fogged. Al waved to us as soon as we were in the door. Next to him stood a petite woman with freckles and a thin smile that nevertheless showed her dimples.

I shook her hand and said "Miss Boston I presume?" to which she replied "Yes, you may call me Alex. Short for Alexandra."

She listened politely while the three of us talked about some of the events. I could picture her and Al as a couple – Al being boisterous and Alex being a steady influence. *Al and Alex. Cute.* She and Al would soon travel overland to Lhasa and other holy sites in Tibet. The pizza was excellent. The crust was just like in Boston's North End and worth every penny. Dessert was ice cream. My share of the bill was more than eleven hundred rupees, which would have been enough to buy a plate of *dal-bhaat* for fifteen people in Tansen.

It was easy to find a taxi to go back to Patan but we were careful to ask whether the driver was on the meter or off. We found one who agreed to go by the meter, which meant no haggling and no gouging. As the taxi drove back to Pulchowk, Padma and I talked again about how we each cried when we left Tansen. I told her she was like the third daughter I never had. When we got home, the neighborhood was dark and candles were lit in the Guest House because the power was out – a rolling blackout. *Seemed like old times.* We said our goodbyes with a quick hug and handshake. She left at four o'clock the following morning to take a bus to India. I got up at five, my usual time, and found a small bag on my doorknob. In it was a note, a final goodbye. "My time in Tansen was richer because of you," she wrote. And a small gift of Cadbury's chocolate.

Boudhanath

Soon after reading Padma's note, I was out the door headed to the thoroughfare near the Eastern Stupa where the taxis parked and waited. I negotiated a fare of three hundred rupees to Boudhanath and hopped in behind a sleepy driver. Out the window I could see people hurrying by with *puja* plates. All the temples in Patan were open. Bells clanged randomly as offerings were made. Kathmandu is sedate at that time of day and we made great time. I arrived at Boudha in the pre-dawn twilight.

At first I walked around the main shrine, but the sounds of chanting echoed from somewhere and I stopped to follow the sound. There was an open gate, and through it I could see an open door and twinkling lights in the early morning dimness. It was a *gompa*, a monastery, and the chanting was morning *puja*, in front of a thirty-foot-high golden statue of Buddha. I took off my tevas and tiptoed in. I sat with my back against the wall and watched the scene. There were a hundred monks in saffron robes. The older monks were in the front row, and the back row was for the very young monks. Six monks played traditional instruments and drums as the rest chanted. The effect was mesmerizing, nonstop sounds that washed back and forth like waves at the edge of a great sea. I thought back to chanting at the Tibetan temple in Honolulu with the two *lamas* that lived there. In Honolulu we never could quite achieve the full effect, and maybe we never would. The chanting continued until nine that morning, with only short breaks as the monks ate their bread with butter tea. During the two hours that I listened, I dozed off a few times and was carried by the sounds – floating somewhere – near the shore.

The monks ended the morning *puja* after three hours, and dispersed. I watched them for a bit, then stood in the doorway to put on my sandals and watch the sun hitting the *stupa*. The *stupa* at Boudhanath is the largest in the world, a five-story mound more than a hundred meters across. The track around it is paved with cobblestones, set in a circular plaza with storefronts that open onto the plaza. Many of the buildings have rooftop restaurants, and there are wild monkeys that live at rooftop. No vehicles are allowed on the plaza. The plaza is not visible from the main road nearby. Visitors must walk through an alley, and then the view of the *stupa* opens up suddenly. It is visible from miles away, but paradoxically from fifty meters away outside, it is hidden by the adjacent buildings. I could not help but think that it was a large human breast with a golden nipple. The Boudhanath Stupa is white and achingly brilliant when the sun shines. Eyes are painted on the spire, and bright prayer flags from all sides in red, blue, yellow, white and green.

The activity at Boudhanath is to walk in circles around the *stupa,* over and over again. Clockwise. This is called *Kora,* and the simple act of walking this route, regardless of your mood or thoughts, is said to bring merit for a future life. At all times during the day there are people doing *Kora.* The most crowded times are in the morning and late afternoon, when there will be hundreds of people walking clockwise, often in groups. On a rainy day there may be fewer people but they will bring a moving forest canopy of umbrellas. The walkers include many women, old and young, in traditional Tibetan costume – many, many Tibetans, maybe an old person in the company of younger relatives, tourists with backpacks, the young single ones, or else tour groups from Italy or other parts of Europe. It seems out of place to see Italian women with short skirts and revealing skintight tank tops, along side Tibetan women in wool, monks in saffron robes, often spinning a prayer wheel as they go, regular people on their way to work.

Many tourists simply walk around the *stupa* a few times without meditating, and call it good. It is an interesting and pleasant tourist site. But I thought back to my retreat with the *Rinpoche* and I was amazed to see how it represented the key teachings of Buddhism. Each trip around the *stupa* is symbolic of one lifetime. When a person walks at the usual speed, they are in the company of roughly the same group of people each time around the *stupa,* forming a *sangha.* Of the walkers nearby, some will inevitably drop off and others may get added each time around. A person who steps off the track and sits on a park bench for awhile will see others disappear, go round the bend, and come back. Climb to a higher level and the circle is smaller. Look down and see the pattern. Contemplate the meaning of *sangha* in your life. The cycle repeats after each person has walked about three-hundred-and-fifteen meters.

I simply walked for two hours, thinking of nothing. Then I stopped for coffee on a rooftop restaurant on the west side of the plaza. I was disappointed to discover that it was instant coffee, but I sipped it anyway. It was unusual to get brewed coffee in Nepal. I unzipped my daypack to get out my guidebook. There was the little colorful silk bag. I thought back to my picnic with Celeste the day before I left for Nepal. I remembered sitting at the picnic table in Waikiki near where she lived, smiling. She had slid the little bag across the table and spilled out the prayer beads.

"I can't give you a gift that costs a lot of money but these have their own value if you know how to use them. Take these and meditate with them in Nepal. This trip will be a transformative experience for you."

That seemed so ironic now. I thought again of the smile of Kusmati's mother, the Magar woman whose baby had such burns, and wondered about Celeste. Celeste with her own private and contradictory ways. *Celeste did not have control of her own life, but she told me I would be transformed.* Now as I took the beads out I thought of touching her hand that day. The beads were light and still smelled of incense. I rubbed them in my hands, warming them to release the oils that would brighten the aroma and pressed them to my forehead as she had done when she gave them to me.

I finished the coffee and put the beads in my pocket. I left a tip and went down the stairs to ground level, past a place that sold Tibetan CDs. On impulse I saw something nice and bought it for Celeste. I decided to make seven *Koras* in a row, one at each level until I got to the highest spot on the *stupa* that still had a usable path. By this time the sun was shining, and a Tibetan woman was feeding handfuls of juniper leaves into the two-meter-tall incense burner on the south side of the *stupa*. An aromatic cloud of burning juniper, like pine needles, billowed over the scene like it was a steam locomotive. *We were burning a bushel of industrial strength incense today.* Earlier I just walked, taking it all in, but this time I found myself thinking about all the people I had met that summer, which naturally led me to think about the ones who had dropped out of sight on the path for now – the ones who had died.

With a start, I thought I recognized a resemblance in the face of one the people walking near me. First one, then another seemed to be right here walking nearby, healthy this time. I suppose it was just the fact that I was seeing people from the same gene pool, and my mind was playing tricks on me, but it seemed a bit spooky. My mind was pre-occupied by feelings of sadness once again. I was still grieving, but like Padma I was now grieving the fact that I was not with the people still working in Tansen, that I had somehow been cut loose. I felt a release of emotion as I contemplated that the Tansen journey was over, a complete event, and one which would now have an end. *Or would it.* I thought about the suffering that took place, all the suffering that was still taking place. *And I was here, not there.* As I walked, I took deep breaths and the tears flowed. I was near the highest level of the *stupa*. Sunlight reflected upwards from the whitewashed dome upon which I stood, and I felt the heat of it. The light from below made the prayer flags stretched overhead seem even brighter as they fluttered in the breeze. I could see three people nearby tug at each others' sleeve as they gestured toward me. They veered off in a different direction so as not to be so close, looking back over their shoulder.

I put my hand in my pocket and touched the beads. Ahead were two women side-by-side, their backs to me, each with long black hair, and again I was startled to think that *there was Celeste, walking side-by-side with Kusmati's mother* as I took my own steps. "*Transformative experience.*" I wished that Celeste was there with me so I could ask her in person about transformative experiences. I wondered if she herself had ever had such a time for her own growth, or if she was just going in circles, *how did she get to that place in her life? What exactly was transformation?* Knowing what I knew now I wanted to go back in time and ask, "*Please list for me the exact ways in which you think I need to be transformed at this present time, and give me a more specific benchmark to use to determine when the transformation is sufficiently complete.*"

Celeste did not know the way any better than I did, she was projecting an aura of wisdom to hide her own insecurity and that was all. I would keep these beads, but it was time to move on with my life and let go of Celeste, just as I had let go of my former wife. *Stop going in circles.* Let go of the anger and volatility that Celeste brought to her world. Let go of drama. Find love instead. And just exist in the world.

I returned to Patan on the bus. When I was almost at the Guest House I noticed a guy standing at a steel fifty-five-gallon drum outside the door of a small Nepali restaurant. He was making *roti*, handling each piece like pizza dough, and then slapping them onto the thick clay lining of the steel drum, a *tandoori* oven. The *roti* looked delicious. That evening, as for most evenings that followed, I returned there to eat. Along with fresh *roti* there was mutton curry. I ordered in Nepali and did not use a utensil. I ate with my right hand. *It's all in the thumb.* I could eat a satisfying meal for a hundred rupees. The spices made the *achaar* intriguing and the *roti* were every bit as good as I hoped. I asked for a spoon, and used it to eat curd (yogurt) for dessert.

The Week in Kathmandu

The week in Kathmandu passed quickly. The dog barked the first night. I found out that if I turned off the entryway light at the Guest House, the dog next door would not bark at all. Each day I was up at five to make coffee and eat bread and fruit. I walked through Patan each day at dawn and I was struck by the degree to which every citizen seemed to take pains to show outward manifestations of Hindu or Buddhist devotion. Women hurried by carrying copper *puja* plates early in the morning, to the temples bustling with incense and energy. On the sidewalks I noticed small wet spots every few yards, sometimes over a brass lotus embedded in the sidewalk, sometimes just on an otherwise unremarkable spot. At these places there was also a bit of red paste, a flower, and a small piece of burned incense – signs of early morning *Puja*. I concluded that I should watch where I put my feet and not step on these since it might be disrespectful.

The day after Padma left, a group of four pastors from Ohio arrived at the Guest House. I asked them their denomination and they said, "Christian." They came to Nepal to speak to a conference about servant leadership in the Christian church of Nepal. The pastors brought donated toys and delivered them to an orphanage. They painted a school house with their hosts. Each day at five I set the breakfast table for them. I made more coffee than usual, filling their thermos with the leftover coffee after I had finished mine, which they appreciated. One morning I offered to take them for a short walk in the neighborhood to see what the morning *puja* was like, but they politely declined. The American pastors were in a bubble set up for them by their Nepali hosts.

I continued my plan to visit the main sites. It was a surprise to see the number of Hindus making *puja* on the grounds of Swayamabunath, the Buddhist *stupa* on a hill overlooking the entire valley. As I approached the stairs to the *stupa*, I passed a series of small, open-fronted shops where old people stooped, rubbing brightly colored pieces of cloth on stone tablets. They were making prayer flags, one at a time, by hand. I climbed the stairs, and enjoyed the panoramic view. Soon I found the reason for all the Hindus to be there. Just behind the *stupa* is the Hindu temple devoted to Sitala, the goddess of smallpox. In typical Hindu logic, Sitala also becomes the goddess who can grant relief to people who are ill from any cause. I sat nearby to watch the *puja* offered by anxious parents on behalf of their sick children, asking for a blessing and the mercy of the Goddess.

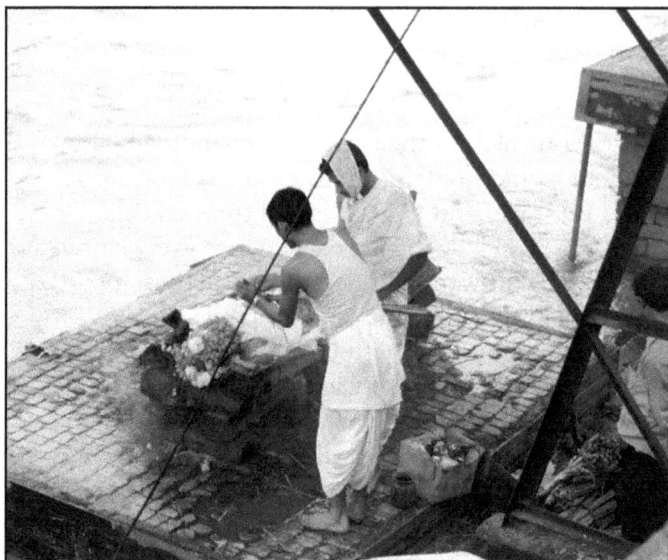

Pashupattinath. The Bagmati River runs through Kathmandu and is a tributary of the Ganges. Funerals here are public events. Here the priest is assisting the first-born son to light the pyre. At the end of the cremation, the ashes will be swept into the river.

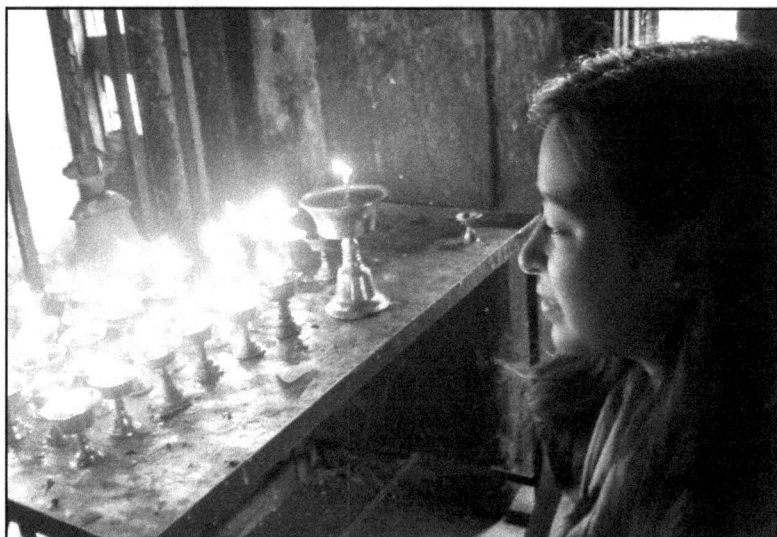

At Sangkhu. The daughter of the temple priest who showed me around. She can trace her heritage back 450 years. Once every four years, every priest's family lives at the temple for a week, a great honor. There was a tray of offertory candles and I donated rupees for the big one since she had given me such a wonderful tour.

The heart of Old Kathmandu is a neighborhood named Ason Tole, which has one of the highest population densities in the world. I walked there for a day, jostled by the crowds and the vitality. I used my guidebook to look for the Toothache Shrine and to my surprise, I found it. Quite by accident, I ran into Matt, "the missionaries minister," and sipped coffee with him at a place in Thamel that reminded me of Starbucks. He told me to start writing.

I visited Bhaktapur on a Monday. It was the day of a festival celebrating Parvati, the wife of Shiva. The square outside the temple was filled by two-thousand women in red saris. There was live music. Street vendors sold those little puff balls with the spicy fillings and I ate some even though I could see that they did not wash their hands. The women were getting *mehandhi*, making small offerings to various *sadhus*, giving money to the beggars lined up outside the temple, and singing. It was hot, but a huge pile of incense was burning in the square outside the temple, which made it even hotter and sent up a choking cloud of aromatic smoke. I recognized women from the same group of Italian tourists that were at Boudhanath a day or two earlier.

Pashupattinath is the place of the cremation *ghats*, said to be second only to Varanasi in holiness as a place for Hindus to move to the next life. This temple is located on the Bagmati River, a tributary of the Ganges, symbolic of the river of human existence. I considered just avoiding this temple altogether but finally decided the experience might be cathartic for me. I arrived on the outskirts just as a crowd of a hundred Shiva pilgrims assembled from an air conditioned chartered bus. They lined up in a procession to approach the temple, wearing saffron yellow T-shirts that said *Shiva Tour 2007* and singing a beautiful hymn in Hindi. After a guided tour I spent the day meditating while the funeral pyres consumed the mortal remains of a dozen different people, delivered one at a time.

One person was cremated on the same *ghat* used to cremate the Royal Family in 2001. To use this *ghat* the family pays a higher fee, so it was a wealthy person. As they washed the body at the riverside, a woman knelt in the shallow water and kissed the feet of the dead person. The next task was to bring the body to the pyre, and as they lifted it, the pallbearers slipped on the terraced steps of wet stone, momentarily juggling the body, then more careful as they carried it over to the neatly stacked wood that waited on the *ghat*. Three-hundred onlookers crowded around, spilling over onto the small stone bridge that crosses the river just downstream. As the fire was lit, the crowd of relatives and friends moved to the shade of the building, men waiting on one side, and women together on the other. In Tansen, women would not have been present.

When lunchtime came, I walked downstream to sit across the river from the less expensive *ghats*. A group of Nepali workmen joined me in the shade of the wall nearby; they were laughing and joking at first. On the other side of the river where the ghats were located, a pickup truck pulled up and a crowd of people unloaded a shrouded body. Then a new funeral started. It was evidently that of a young woman. A young child mournfully called out ,"Aaaaaaamaaaa!" and it seemed as though a zone of silence spread like ripples after the kerplunk of a pebble dropped into water. Each time the toddler repeated the cry, calling for her mother, the ripples of silence spread a little further until I felt as though I could hear a pin drop fifty meters away. I did not notice the sound of the birds overhead 'til now. *Aama!*

The husband, a young man, needed to be supported by two other young men, maybe his brothers, as he walked around the pyre three times with the flaming torch. The men on either side steadied him as he lit the fire, gazing on his lover's face for the last time. The workmen that were joking became silent now; any sense of bravado had dissipated along with the smoke across the river. The two that were smoking stubbed their cigarettes out. We could see the husband sob as his head was shaved while he sat on the stone steps by the water. The two friends also sat while the barber shaved their heads, then the three men held each other and wept. From a distance we did not know the name or the circumstances. The workmen on my side of the river stood up quietly, shook the stiffness out of their legs, and left. *Namaste.* I felt emotionally spent.

Changu Narayan is in the countryside, further away than Bhaktapur. The next morning after my trip to Pashupattinath, I got to the taxi stand early. The head guy told me to get into one particular taxi, but it would not start. Three other drivers were press-ganged into pushing the taxi to jump start it, and it still would not go, and I thought of getting out, but they kept at it and for a minute I wondered if they would push me all the way to Changu. They literally pushed the taxi for about a half mile as if they were a bobsled team. The engine turned over and caught. As we picked up speed I looked back to see the pushers all flop down right in the middle of the road, heaving for breath. I told the driver not to wait for me while I visited the temple.

I walked up the hill to the temple through the small, tidy brick town, listening to the early morning devotional concert of Krishna music broadcast over a loudspeaker. At first I thought it was a recording, but in a room on the same floor as the temple courtyard was a six-piece live band, seated in an enclosure of chicken wire, talking and joking between songs. No other westerners around. I sat and talked with a man from the town who pulled a folded-up leaf from his pocket. In it was an aromatic paste, which he called *Chandan*.

"This tree grows right here and this is the tika of Changu."

He smeared a small dot of it on my forehead, giving a dash of color over my third eye. He then told me that instead of returning via Bhaktapur, I should go to Sangkhu to see the temple there. We stood on a vantage point where the route to get to Sangkhu could be seen as if on a map.

A van load of tourists arrived, just as the band was packing up their instruments. I recognized the same group of Italians that had followed me every day so far. Their guide walked them methodically through the sculptures for which Changu is famous, stopping to describe each one. The Italian women wore tank tops which revealed every contour of their torso, leaving nothing to the imagination, a sharp contrast to the modesty of rural Nepal. On the grounds of Changu is a small shrine to Kali, the fierce feminine goddess of destruction. Morning *puja* was now over and the Kali temple was closed, but the sun was rising and the heat was bearing down, so the Italian women sat in a line under the shady eaves of the shrine, passing a water bottle along. *I wonder what Kali would think of the tank tops*, I thought as I took their photo. Changu is at the end of a long ridge with a panoramic view on three sides. After Changu, I returned through the town but veered off away from the road, down the hill, through the rice paddies, following the narrow dikes which meandered between paddies. *Why not take the man's advice and see the temple of Tara, the Goddess. Celeste will enjoy this story.* The rice was chest high and the heads were getting full. I kept my eye out for snakes and there were none. *It would have been ironic to get bitten now.* Next I rolled up my pant legs to ford a small stream then climbed up an embankment to get to the road where I could catch a bus to Sangkhu.

The town was surrounded by flooded rice paddies as if it were an island. On the green wooded hillside above the town you could see the golden spires and prayer flags of the Vajra Yogini temple. I picked my way through the streets in the general direction. Resting dogs would lift up their head as I went by. They seemed mellow. *Maybe the dogs of Sangkhu are Buddhists.* I arrived at the long stairs to the temple and found that I had again leapfrogged with the Italians. They were climbing back into their van as I arrived. They watched as I spoke to their guide in Nepali. He told me the Italians were headed to Tibet the next day. I asked him whether he thought the Tibetans would enjoy the tank tops. He laughed and said *Ke garne?* ("What is there to do?"). I continued up the stairs.

The temple was open for afternoon *puja*; I walked up alongside townspeople carrying large platters with mounds of *bhaat* and sliced fruit.

A uniformed security guard was there, posted to prevent picture-taking. I wandered around for a bit, careful about the horde of wild monkeys that swarmed all around. Somebody asked me what I thought about the temple and I answered in Nepali, which surprised them so a small crowd gathered. My Nepali language was still not the best, but when the people at the temple discovered I was a University Professor, the wife of the priest summoned their daughter who could speak English and who wanted to study in the US. Soon I was being given a personal tour. The daughters led me up the hill to the chamber of the "upper Goddess," in whose presence we sat for a half hour. As we entered the room, we showed respect by kneeling momentarily to touch our foreheads to a brass lotus embedded in the floor, covered with red *tika* powder. Then we sat silently for a while in the presence of the Goddess, a large brass statue, adorned with a red dress. *She wears it because she is a woman and wants to look nice.* The afternoon included drinking *chiya* with the family in their personal quarters nearby while I gave the daughter college advice. I did not know of any scholarship help for her but I think she appreciated the advice I gave about how to contact private colleges.

The daughters told me about the Goddess of that particular temple and how she protected the town. For them, Buddhism was inseparable from the Goddess. As they accompanied me back to the stairs, we stopped to see the cave carved from the solid rock where people formerly would fast and meditate for months at a time.

They told me, "If a person is holy enough they can get out of the cave even though the door is locked."

Then a local guy, evidently holy enough, demonstrated the secret of the cave which unlocked that mystery. According to another legend, if a person stays in the cave for twenty-four hours without eating or drinking, their prayers will be granted.

On the way back to Kathmandu, I took the public bus. To get back to Patan I needed to make two transfers, one of which involved jumping onto the back bumper of a slow-moving *tuk-tuk*. The vehicle accelerated unexpectedly while I was half-on, half-off. I banged my shin so bad I almost let go and fell off, but two Nepali guys who were already on the back bumper platform reached around me until I was steady. They hugged me and shouted words of encouragement as I held on for dear life, gripping the bar with one hand as pain shot up my leg, steadying myself on the back bumper and rubbing my shin with the other hand as the *tuk-tuk* sped up. Right behind me, also accelerating, was a car that was so close it would have run me over as soon as I fell off. When I got to Patan I limped home.

I was ready to leave Nepal. The night before I got on the plane, I got to the last page of my journal. I thought about the bubble again, and I wondered about the difference between the God of the *New Testament* and the God of the *Old Testament*. Maybe the nature of God could change depending on where you were in your personal bubble. The trip was finished and there were no pages left in the journal. The last word I wrote was *Pugio*.

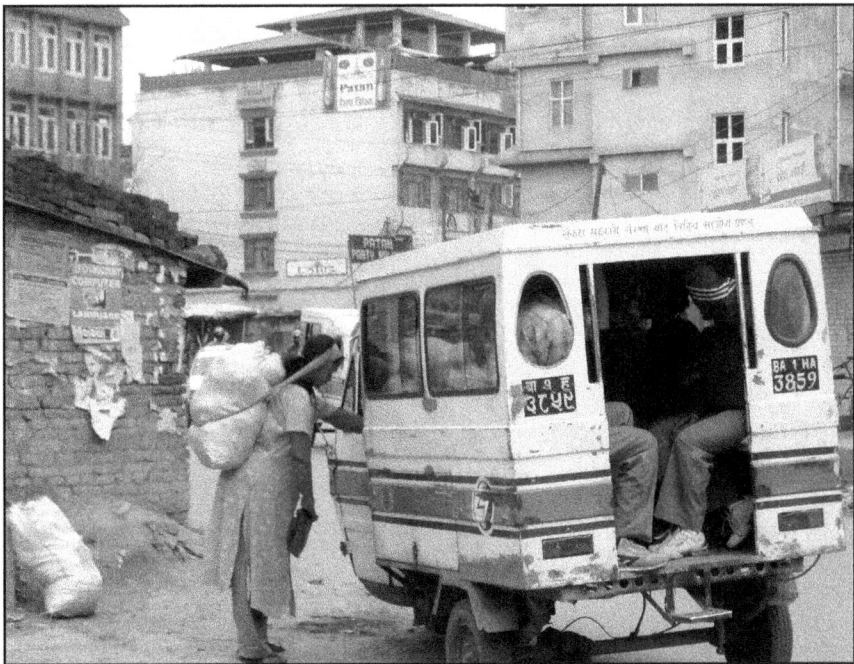

A *tuk-tuk* in Patan. Note the Woman with the pack-basket or *Dhoka*. I rarely rode on these after the day I nearly fell off the back bumper of one.

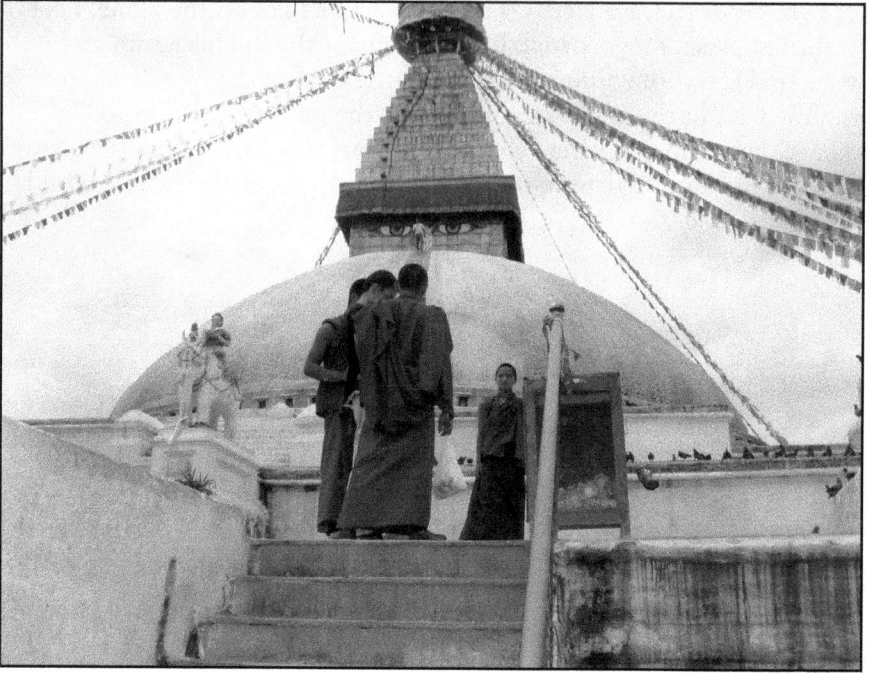

At Boudhanath. What exactly is transformation?

What I Missed

It was not until after I returned to the US that I heard about the bus accident. I got the news from two sources. In this day and age news travels quickly around the globe, and you can hear instantly of all catastrophes. This accident did not make the headlines anywhere, which is a measure of Tansen's isolation.

I do not know the details of the actual accident, but at Mission Hospital, the first vehicles arrived with no advance notice. Bleeding victims tumbled out. More and more came. The ER staff decided to initiate a full-fledged disaster process. The first step was to call the *Chowkidars* to herd a hundred people out of the large waiting room so that it could be used as a triage and treatment area. Nursing students and all off-duty doctors were assembled, and the large box with casualty supplies was opened so that equipment and supplies were readily available. There were eight deaths. Thirty-two people were admitted and many were sent to Theater for emergency surgery. There was chaos and suffering along with hard work by the health workers.

The accident did not make the American news. One of the Nepali interns at Mission Hospital emailed me about it, and a Nepali graduate student at the University also got an email from his family.

It actually happened while I was still in Kathmandu. I was already gone from Tansen just prior to this because I knew I needed time in Kathmandu to recover before returning to Hawaii for the start of fall semester. If I had stayed another week, 'til the last possible minute, I would have been there the day it happened.

When I heard about it, I told the story of the accident to a faculty colleague who had taught nursing in Samoa for fifteen years. She looked at me and she said, "But deep down in your heart you wish you had stayed the extra week and been there, don't you? Admit it, its okay to say so."

And it was true. *I wished I had been there.* I would have worked my butt off. There was a piece of me that wanted to work with the team one more time. There was a piece of me that would do anything for those people. There was a piece of me that would have loved the excitement. There was a piece of me that would have dreaded the suffering. There was a piece of me that was glad I missed it. There was a piece of me that wondered whether I would have finally, truly, and irrevocably cracked the day after. Here in Honolulu, there was a faculty colleague who could see these pieces and help me put the puzzle back together again.

Return to Honolulu

My last connection was in Tokyo and I boarded the plane with several large Japanese tour groups wearing name tags, dressed in designer jeans and lots of leather. I sat next to a honeymoon couple that looked like they were eighteen years old. She was poring through shopping advertisements. In Tokyo I looked around for a woman, any woman, wearing a *sari*. I saw only Japanese women, and the odd American. This was a signal to take off my *topi* and fold it before putting it in the daypack. I slept on the flight.

It was a bright morning in Honolulu when the plane touched down. It was easy to get through Customs, and I took a taxi home. My parents greeted me with hugs and kisses. They made coffee while I unpacked. As we drank it, I gave my mom a red *pashmina* shawl and a *potey*, the green beaded necklace the married ladies wore. I told them about the guy who had been bitten by the snake. My dad asked a lot of good questions about ventilation and wanted the specifics of the electrical problem as I thought he might.

After I answered his questions I thanked him for dragging me along on all those home repair projects. "You taught me things I never learned in nursing school."

Then I told them about the woman who kissed my hand, and I gave my dad the *topi* I wore the week I took care of Dharsha. Mom and dad were proud of me and tears came to their eyes. My dad told me in his usual loud voice that in early July he was worried that I might have joined a cult of some kind and never return. I told him I needed my teaching job, especially the health insurance. I told them I was glad to be back, but even as I said it I knew it wasn't exactly true. *As to whether I might return to Nepal –*

Mom made lunch, BLT sandwiches, and they were exactly the way she made them when I was a kid. *Remarkable.* My dad proudly reported that he had accomplished his goal: he rode every single bus line on Oahu over the course of the summer.

I said, "Okay, if you are so smart, how would you get from here to – Waianae?"

Without batting an eyelash he said, "That's easy, take the five or the six to Ala Moana, then get on the forty or the forty A. Or maybe the C Express. You're going to have to do better than that if you want to stump me."

He could rattle of the bus numbers with authority. I thought maybe I should call the TV station or do something to memorialize the accomplishment. *Now there was something to keep you busy. He was working on his quest when I was working on mine. At least he was smart enough to include a definite end point.* They enjoyed the trip to Maui even though they mistakenly took Route 30, the cliffside road that approaches Lahaina from the north, and it scared them to death. They loved Waikiki. "I felt like I was in another, more beautiful world," said my mom.

"I know that feeling," I replied.

The trade winds made the weather here so much more bearable than if my parents had stayed for the humid thunderstorms of South Florida. They sent dozens of postcards to all their friends in Florida.

In the airport at Tokyo there had been a place sponsored by Yahoo Dot Com that offered free internet access so I parked myself there for awhile to kill time. I read an email from Celeste offering to pick me up at the airport but I replied to say I was okay. I did not phone Celeste until after my parents were on the plane to Florida and when I finally did, she sounded abrupt. Too busy to make time for me. No explanation. A few days later she called and said she was ready to hear the stories. I invited her for dinner. I made lamb while she tried on a *cholo* with a *patuka*. We held hands across the table and shared a moment of silence. The first story I wanted to tell her was about the Magar woman and her daughter, but I felt hurried and I could not find the words to convey the emotional impact. I was just not articulate enough. She wanted to get to the punch line as if it could be neatly wrapped up with a bow. The story trailed off into nowhere. We changed topics.

After we ate, Celeste fretted about the DUI arrest. She would not go into details. I had no idea what the penalty might be. I was surprised when she told me it was a felony. She was relying on the public defender because she could not afford a lawyer. She switched into a tone of voice I had not heard from her since the first weeks we met. *She was using the crackling oat bran voice on me.* And at first I blushed. *Maybe* – but then I listened carefully to what she was actually saying. She was having financial worries and she needed three-thousand dollars. She cleared her throat and wondered if there was a way I could co-sign a loan for her to tidy up some bills. I asked her if she had any credit of her own and she said, "no." She could not get a loan by herself any more. It was a long story as to how it happened to be that way.

I looked at Celeste for a long second, thinking about Kusmati's mother and the times in Nepal I had thought about the sound of Celeste's voice and the way she smiled. And now she was across my kitchen table with the red-checkered tablecloth and a candle between us. *You know I would do anything for you,* I wanted to say. After a pause I told her I needed to deal with my own cash flow and I did not have an answer for her, not now, maybe next week. Her face turned red and her attitude shifted to more nervous fidgeting. We kept talking about the events of the summer but there was a hollow feeling, as we tried to fill the space. Soon I could see that she was growing anxious and trying to control her anger. There were some periods of silence, and we could both sense the tension. Celeste cut the evening short and left. Two hours later I was awakened by the cell phone. I picked it up without looking to see who it was. She was apologetic and sweet, trying to rebuild bridges. *Maybe she did want to hear about how I felt.* But I still did not lend her money.

At Boudhanath, I got Celeste a present on the spur of the moment, spending more than I wanted, thinking it was still worth it. I wrapped it carefully for the trip, and set it aside when I got home. I still have it, out of the box. Sometimes it reminds me of her, but since I never saw her with it, there are other times when it reminds me mostly of my own frame of mind when I just finished a major chapter of my life.

People kept telling me I was thinner, so I finally weighed myself and I was fifteen pounds lighter. I went to my regular doctor and got a stool test for Ova and Parasites. *Negative. Not a critter to be seen.* Another TB test. *Negative.*

In September I was at a UH School of Nursing faculty committee meeting and we were discussing some policy that might address an anticipated student problem when I blurted, "We don't have to put up with bullshit." Heads turned.

A colleague said, "Is that Joe? Doesn't sound like you? Joe, what has got into you?"

People told me I seemed so somber nowadays and I knew that I needed to work on re-entry, getting used to being back in Hawaii. Once school got into full swing, I resumed supervising UH students in clinical practice at a local hospital. One morning, one of the older students took me aside to say that when I was humming, *Tell Me Why*, she could tell I was far away and not having a good day.

"What happened to you there, Joe?" she asked. I was momentarily stunned by the degree of sensitivity this showed. *She was right, of course.*

I gave a couple of talks to the UH nursing students about my experience. I made a PowerPoint presentation that consisted of pictures, no captions. There were no statistics to memorize. People could just take in the images as I spoke. When I showed it to our community health nursing class, I started out by asking for two volunteers and dressing them in the costumes I brought home, complete with tassels and *patukas*. The class loved it. Then we got serious as the pictures were displayed. I focused on Pediatrics. The students could see the people, the hospital, and the town. I could talk about the communicable diseases and the dedicated staff. Finally I got to the pictures of burn victims, including Padma's photo of the baby with the head burn. Even with forewarning there was a collective gasp when they saw the photo of the baby with the burn on her buttocks. I thought, *I will revise my slide show before next time. Or maybe not.*

I packed the Magar Hill Woman outfits into boxes and mailed them from Honolulu to my former wife and my two daughters along with detailed instructions as to how to wear each piece. At first they did not know what to do with these items, but finally tried them on. They each told me that they loved the way the *cholo* fit. My guess work on the sizes was accurate after all. My former wife wore her *cholo* to work one day, but left the *patuka* behind. I have spoken with her on the phone since my return, and it was very civil. I told her *Nepal was fine. Someday I will tell you about it.*

Which translates as *Never.*

I had a dream in which I got in the car and went to Honolulu Airport to meet myself coming off the plane. When I got there, I waited among the crowd of greeters in the arrival area. The doors opened and there were happy reunions all around. If I got off the plane, I did not recognize myself. I kept waiting, but as the crowd thinned, I realized that I was not on the plane in the first place. There was a message saying I was still in Nepal. The crowd dissipated and I went home, empty handed. I only had that dream one time.

Doctor Norma emailed in September to say that Kusmati and Akash were improving all the time. People at the University and at church ask me what the trip to Nepal was like and I say, "Fine. Everyone should go."

At church one Sunday the choir sang *Be Thou My Vision.* My eyes got misty. I closed them and pictured myself standing at English-language service among dear friends.

I ran into Celeste by accident in December. She beamed when she saw me, and we talked for a bit. She triumphantly told me that the DUI case had been thrown out on a technicality. She told me she was in love. Her new boyfriend was a cable TV installer who supplemented his income with a part-time job being a DJ at high school and middle school dances. They met in a bar.

"He's not very smart but I have decided that intelligence isn't everything," she said. "He's ten years younger than me too – I never thought I would go for a younger man."

I pictured Celeste sitting proudly with her new guy behind the DJ console on the stage of a school gym somewhere. She asked if I wanted to meet him and I said no. *Celeste as a DJ groupie. Maybe Celeste could dance with the high school kids while he worked.* Celeste blushed when she saw that I could barely suppress my laughter. I wondered if he had any money to lend.

Wrapping It Up

Over the course of writing this manuscript I made a promise to myself to stick to an unsentimental description of the events and facts. I shared not only what I learned but my reaction to events at the time. The trip was not a vacation in the sense of rejuvenation and relaxation, and was considerably more intense and personal than I expected it would be before I began. I literally could not speak about some of these things, and writing was a means to cast light on what would otherwise be a dark corner of my mind. The act of writing brought me serenity. Each reader can ponder for themselves, how they would have reacted or what they might have been thinking had they been in the situation instead of me.

First, for a medical person there is more to the experience than prayer and *Bible* study. Your skills and knowledge are your primary offering to God. The people described in this book all contributed in different ways, some more successfully than others, but for each of them, their skills were the best offering to God they could devise. Some readers may be shocked to learn that missionaries also drink beer or get angry; or that their skills are not enough; or that they are sometimes bored – or that they are human. For those shocked readers, my advice is – get over it. Being human is the essence of life. To try is sometimes to fail.

Next, if any reader with professional-level medical or nursing skills wishes to embark on a similar adventure, my advice is to prepare carefully. Go. Do. Get out from under the Bubble, and find a place to serve, somewhere near "the end of the world." At the beginning of this book I defined the bubble as a set of western comforts and attitudes. The bubble also includes a veneer of fear that envelopes us when we get out into the world. In that sense I succeeded in getting beyond the bubble, and from my position outside it, I can see that the bubble of fear is propagated by what we read, what we see on TV, and hear on the radio. We are saturated with news of Iraq and Afghanistan, or Somalia or the bombings in Mumbai. Even in books, a more subdued part of the media palette, there has to be a villain, depicted as some type of inscrutable or fanatical "other." Be wary of your own notions of a bogeyman. When the media and books reinforce these stereotypes, the resulting fear is amplified to the point where you will stay home. In reality, most of the hazards can be mitigated by careful preparation. I am not saying that everything is wonderful in other parts of the world – indeed, it is not – but I have now written the book I wish had been available before my own trip.

When you come back, share your story. Give yourself time to re-adjust, and realize that you may never truly feel comfortable in the Bubble again. There is value in the mission experience, not just in how we serve, but in what we bring back.

For myself, on a practical level, when I go up and down the aisles at the supermarket, I find that I don't buy such a variety of items any more. The packaging seems like too much waste. My apartment has no clutter since I never buy anything. My meals are much simpler. I never watched much TV before, but now I watch even less. I thought about selling my car and moving to a less expensive apartment.

Of course, you might as well add my name to the long list of people who embark on an adventure, something completely off the wall, right after a divorce. This trip was something I always wanted to do but had put off for one reason or another. Things could have been worse. To my credit, I survived my first post-marriage relationship (if you call it that) with hardly any scars, and I also still have a roof over my head. The experience of living in a foreign culture, immersed in the daily life there, learning about Hinduism and Buddhism, is something I will cherish forever. My ears perk up when I hear the news from South Asia. Now I also have new friends with whom I share things that others do not begin to comprehend. Life goes on, and I am eager to see what is next.

The inner turmoil of dealing with sad situations has passed and I now look back with deep satisfaction on all that I was able to do. Is this the same as being "transformed?" I guess I don't show outward signs of acting "more spiritual." I sometimes think I am the only American to go to Nepal, rich with Hinduism and Buddhism, who ended up praying to the Christian God with every ounce of strength I possessed.

My time outside the bubble made me think about the dedication it takes to deliver health care. In Tansen I saw some very smart people who worked hard to create miracles even though there were limited resources. Here in the US, I see some people who have all the resources in the world but fail to use them. It makes me wonder why they settle for anything less than excellence, and it makes me a bit more willing to prod those around me into better performance. I promised myself that in the US, I would never complain about the equipment any more, but I do find that I demand more from my students when I compare them to their counterparts in Nepal. So I am not in some sort of daily Zen-like trance of peaceful wisdom and acceptance. What would happen here in the West, if everyone treated their daily job as if it were their mission?

I know damn well that there are many more stories out there, and there are also people who did a lot more than I did and stayed longer. Some have returned to their home country. Others are still in Tansen and they are role models to me. I think of those people every day and I want God to bless them for what they do.

On New Year's Eve as I finished writing this story, I noticed that I was happy. Returning to a point where I could feel the joy of being alive again was a gradual process, with no particular turning point. I have a renewed sense of optimism and hope for the world, tempered by the idea that to fix the problems will require an effort by everyone. I will return to Nepal. Maybe not to Tansen. Maybe someplace even more rural, where they need me more. In the meantime, I have concluded that I spent summer 2007 at the finest hospital on planet earth.

Acknowledgements

I interacted with hundreds of people at Tansen, and I can not acknowledge them all, nor can I tell everything in the detail I would like. Shakuntala Thanju, known as "Principal Ma'am" and Sr. Patricia Conroy, M.M., RN, Ph.D., from Tansen Nursing School are two that deserve special mention for their vision and support. At Mission Hospital the medical staff, employees, faculty, and nursing students were wonderful to me.

Members of SNEHA, the Society of Nepalese in Hawaii, were helpful. Bedika Upadhyaya, my tutor in Honolulu, deserves special thanks. Khela Neupane was my Tansen-based language tutor and cultural confidante. Khela, my time in Tansen was richer because of you.

Transliterated spelling from Devanagari to Roman alphabet is not exact. I am indebted to Mandira Neupane (no relation to Khela), a native Nepali speaker, for her review of the transliterations of Nepali words in the glossary of terms, as well as other cultural nuances.

The Director of International Programs at UH School of Nursing, John Casken, was very supportive of this trip, as was Ann Sloat and Mary Boland. Stan and Alicia Niemczura, my parents, lived in my apartment while I was gone. They brought in the mail, kept the grass mowed, tackled some minor home repairs, and addressed a variety of issues. They were the best stateside support team I could have asked for.

Ellen Bridge, Betsy Gettman, Steve Gruverman, Tom Niemczura, Alok Rajouria, Sudha Acharya, and the late Gene Sylvester, read early drafts of this manuscript and provided valuable feedback. Patricia Brooks, my faculty colleague, helped me to reframe my reentry issues and resume a normal life, whatever that is. I am fortunate to be surrounded by talented and dedicated colleagues at the University of Hawaii at Manoa who have served all over the world. Likewise, the students in my fall semester 2007 courses who kept me on track.

They say that producing a book is like having a baby. If the analogy holds, then poet, Susan Bright, my editor, was a gentle midwife. Her motto (a quotation from Meridel LeSueur) is "hard times ain't quit, and we ain't quit". Susan, thank you for the story about your grandmother who was a missionary nurse in Asia. For all intents and purposes, "You had me at hello." The reader is strongly encouraged to browse the Plain View Press website for other works by this fine publishing house. (www.plainviewpress.net)

About the Names

The reader should be alerted to one important concern that provided a dilemma for me while writing. I needed to change the names of some specific major characters from this experience, and to change the details of their lives, physical appearance, and location. The purpose is twofold. First, to protect the privacy of persons who wish to remain out of the public spotlight since they did not know they would be characterized in this work. Second, to mitigate the possibility of a lawsuit.

My thinking is that the superficial identifying characteristics are relatively unimportant to the narrative, and that the meat of the story lies with the things they did or said, as opposed to who exactly they may be. The things they did or said, remain.

Once I decided to change *some* names, I also decided to change the names of *all* the major players, even those who have every reason to be very proud of how they contributed. For the medical missionaries portrayed in this book, their daily medical mission work is their offering to God, and takes on an intensely personal element, which adds to the privacy concerns.

Of course, it is impossible to change the names or identities of the blood relatives mentioned here. I beg their indulgence and forgiveness. The cumulative effect of this is to change the category of the book from "nonfiction" to "creative nonfiction." Be that as it may, the major clinical details, the types of cases and outcomes, and the thrust of the events remain as close to my actual recollection as I can render them.

Appendix 1

What Would Florence Nightingale Do?

Among the medical community of Tansen, there was a saying. "We will know when we are approaching the same indicators of health and illness as the West, when the patients start dying of the same illnesses." The illnesses described in this book are a plague to Nepal and the lesser developed, or war-ravaged, areas of the planet. They would largely disappear if there were clean water, sewage disposal, immunizations,

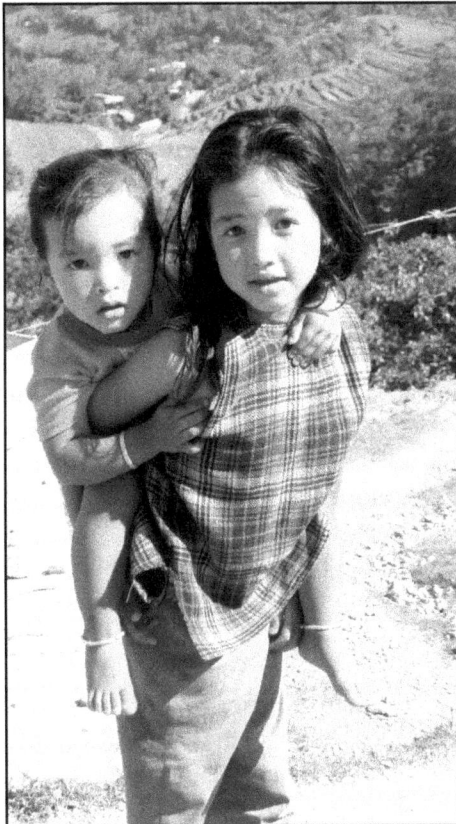

Women in rural Nepal are taught to carry burdens from early in life, whether it is water, fodder, wood, or a younger sibling.

contact follow-up for infectious diseases, availability of contraception, and inspection of meat. To this list, add a better energy system which does not rely on wood and kerosene, regulation of alcohol, and an adequate supply of protein to children. If the one million people in the vicinity of Tansen had these things, there would be a dramatic change in the type of patient to be found in the wards at Mission Hospital. People would lead the lives God planned for them.

Women lead a disproportionately hard life in Nepal. Teen pregnancy, family violence, early widowhood, preferential treatment for boys, unavailability of prenatal care, human trafficking, unsanitary home birth, and lack of contraception are among the issues. Women were among the most ardent Maoists – they were fighting for their health and that of their children.

Nursing is an important part of the solution to all these problems. In the past ten years nursing education has become a clear gateway to a professional role for women in Nepal, beyond that of wife and mother. Nurses in the community become powerful voices and leaders of a better way to care for children, the sick and aged. The leaders of nursing in Nepal know that they are imparting a whole new way for their students to relate to the world. In their society the nursing leaders are radical feminists on par with our own early suffragettes. In the West, it is fashionable for the intelligentsia to brush aside the role of women (and men!) who choose to study nursing as opposed to medicine. This is a huge mistake, and we need to do a better job to respect and support the nurse's role throughout the world. To do this is to honor our mother and the mothers of our children.

We need to re-examine ways for western countries to help nursing education in lesser developed countries. To send the nurses to the US or UK for training is a poor use of resources due to the vast differences in the systems, and one which belies the need to avert a brain drain. The nurses are needed right where they are. Next is to find a way to pay them. It is a paradox that hospitals need nurses, and train them, but can't hire them afterwards due to the poverty of the people being served. Also, the scarcity of textbooks can hardly be overstated. The books that I brought to Nepal will be in use long after I am dead. Why not find a way to send more teachers from the US? Why not a national effort in the US to supply better text books and teachers to these countries? Why not find better funding for the international nursing organizations that could lift up the role of women everywhere? Why not?

Appendix 2

Within the Walls of the Hospital Compound

The average American might picture Mission Hospital as a collection of thatched-roof huts in a jungle clearing. It is not that way at all. There is a walled compound with guards. Inside the wall is a collection of brick buildings from different eras over the past fifty years. The hospital started small and added a wing here and there over time. It is a mile from the *Bajar* in Tansen, originally surrounded by meadows. But over the course of time a small community of hotels and restaurants grew up just outside the hospital gates, forming an urban neighborhood in the immediate vicinity. The street directly in front of the hospital is paved for about a hundred yards, on either end of the paved section it is gravel.

The hospital owns a variety of kinds of equipment. The Operating Theater is air-conditioned. The hospital is proud of their C-arm X-Ray machine and the ultrasound machine. The Clinical staff is supported by a fully equipped lab and blood bank. Mission Hospital can perform a caesarean delivery in fifteen minutes. They can administer thrombolytic drugs and give modern anesthesia. There is a clinic in Butwal that owns a CT scan, and patients from Mission Hospital can go there to get a CT scan. It is expensive but at least it is available.

Mission Hospital employs more than three-hundred people. The Chief Executive Officer oversees a pyramidal hierarchy of department heads. The policy manual is updated regularly. The bureaucracy parallels that of a hospital in the US. Just down the hill is a nursing school that enjoys an excellent reputation. The Non-Governmental Organization (NGO) that operates Mission Hospital has been in Nepal for fifty years and also runs other hospitals, but Tansen is the oldest.

Mission Hospital has a very active community health service. This includes an off campus Maternal-Child Clinic; a Nutritional Resource Center; clinics in outlying areas; and preventative programs. These are absolutely critical to the mission, but I have not written about them because I was not involved in them. The work of public health is not as dramatic as the day-to-day events of acute care. Material for a future book I suppose.

There are various estimates as to the "catchment area" of the hospital. For a lay person, this is roughly the number of people in the geographic area who would consider the hospital to be the place where they would go if they were sick. The estimates range from 250,000 to

1,000,000 people. Now, ask yourself this question. If there was just one 160-bed hospital for a population of 1,000,000 people, what would it be like? Who would be in the beds?

There are quite a few things Mission Hospital does not have. This is where it gets interesting. In some cases, this is because the administration made a conscious choice about cost-effective services given the limited resources. I respect the choices made by the administration there. The circumstances are difficult and I believe they have acted with the highest possible ethical standard.

There is a well-established Missionary community at Tansen, almost two-dozen adults and a variety of kids. The mission kids attend a one-room schoolhouse on the grounds with a teacher from Canada. The family life is best described as "wholesome."

Mission Hospital is now a major training site for the Nick Simons Institute, an NGO which seeks to improve the professional medical knowledge of the Nepali people so that they do not rely so much on foreigners. Mission Hospital is also a site for Nepali interns and residents in a cooperative program headquartered in Kathmandu.

A number of years ago, some of the Missionary Medical staff at Tansen produced a reference book which they named the *Tansen Guidelines*. This book, now out of print, described a decision making process for clinical care in Nepal. Because Mission Hospital has been considered to be a model hospital, the Guidelines were distributed to the other hospitals in the UMN network and served as a basis for treatment decisions. Over the course of time this added to the reputation of Tansen.

Finally, it should be noted that UMN has been the beneficiary of tremendous charity support over the years, and the facility has many plaques and memorials to the organizations that have provided major gifts. These are as diverse as Lions International, a Netherlands agency for international development, and Mossley Parish Church, in Newtonabbey, Northern Ireland.

Appendix 3

Learning the Nepali Language

There are no nursing textbooks written in the Nepali language, and throughout the country nurses and doctors are taught using the English language. Our students studied from books published in India or Kathmandu, printed on cheap paper with no color plate illustrations. A typical American textbook costs more than three month's wages for an adult Nepali, and no student could own a personal textbook. The students always studied in groups. That is why the school wanted American textbooks. When they opened the seven boxes of books, two employees spent three days cataloging them, and assigned them a value of twelve thousand US dollars for accounting purposes. They were very grateful and this gift created a lot of goodwill. The school owned several computers and they especially liked the books that came with CDs.

Even though the students were bilingual I decided to learn the Nepali language before I got there. I figured it would help me get out from under the bubble. I called the University of Hawaii language department to ask about taking a course in Nepali. No, they did not offer coursework in this language. No, they did not know of anybody who could teach me either. I was on my own to find a private tutor. *Now here is an interesting puzzle.* To solve it, I made a small flyer that said, *UH Professor seeks a Nepali language tutor.* There is just one Indian grocery store in Honolulu and it is located near the University. I walked down one Saturday and spoke to the man behind the counter. He smiled and posted my little flyer next to the Bollywood DVDs. Within six hours I got a phone call. The woman was originally from Kathmandu and her husband was a UH graduate student. She would teach me and we arranged weekly lessons.

Each week I would go to my tutor's apartment and sit with my tutor on a sheet spread on the living room floor for the lesson while her six-year-old daughter watched. The family also ate while sitting cross-legged on a sheet spread out in the living room. My knees would get tired and sooner or later I would move to the easy chair.

One week my tutor called to remind me not to eat before coming over because we would have dal-bhaat, the staple food that people in Nepal eat at least once a day. There is a steel dish with a high rim around it, and when sit are on the floor to eat, you hold the dish in your lap. On the dish is a mound of cooked rice (bhaat) along with a small bowl of lentil soup (*dal*). Next to it in a separate compartment is some *sag*, green and leafy like cooked spinach. Maybe there are some cucumber slices and a hot pepper or two. Sometimes there will be a little yogurt, sometimes a little mutton curry in a side dish. In the last compartment will be *achaar*, a sort of condiment based on tomatoes with spices. Pour the lentil soup over the rice, and mix it with your right hand, sometimes swirling with the palm. Pick up a ball of rice, with your thumb bent *just so* to keep it steady, and pop it into your mouth. Nepali people can do this neatly. My first time was not so neat. At a restaurant the servers will keep filling up your plate as you eat, unless you tell them you are full, for which the term is *pugio*.

Once the food comes out, people eat without talking, sometimes without even looking up. After eating, water is poured over the right hand to wash it. Nepalis are always curious to see whether a *videshi* will eat the Nepali way, or ask for a spoon. I never saw people linger once the meal was finished. You do your talking before the food comes out. My tutor also made me some *Chiya*, tea the Nepali way. It was strong and I was awake the whole night afterwards.

Learning the language started with the syllabary. This is the linguistic term for the alphabet of Devanagari, in which Nepali is written. It is very similar to Sanskrit, the writing system of northern India. There are thirty three consonants, and eleven vowels. Learning only forty-four characters is not enough. There is a system of eleven diacritical markers that may be placed before or after each consonant to change the sound; and there are "conjunct" characters to learn – a conjunct is when two consonants are squeezed together. Finally, there are about a hundred and fifty "half-characters."

In the languages that use Devanagari, the pronunciation of certain letters does not lend itself well to an American transliteration. There is a subtle "breathiness" which changes some letters. I recall spending a half-hour sitting on the floor trying to master the difference between "ta," "tHa" and "taw," which was interrupted by hysterical laughter.

I made flash cards for the vowels and consonants and carried them with me wherever I went. I practiced every day. Within two months I was getting it. Later, I added flash cards for the simple words I learned. One day during my class with the nursing students I was writing the schedule on the blackboard and said to myself *I wonder how I would spell 'coffee' using Devanagari*. With a moment's thought I was able to come up with the spelling, and stood at the blackboard chuckling. I turned around and I could see the students were not really paying attention. Oh well.

I made a special trip to the bookstore to get a guidebook. I got to the travel section looking for Asia. There they were, five possible guidebooks on Nepal. *Which one to buy?* I flipped through each, looking to see if there was a section on Tansen. The first two only gave it a paragraph. "Nice hill town," was about all they said. *You know you are off the map when it's not in the Lonely Planet.* The guide from the Moon Handbook series included five pages along with a small schematic map. That is the one I bought. I photocopied the pages and posted them outside my office door so that people could see where I was going for the summer.

Appendix 4

What Is Different About Hospitals In Nepal?

The first three weeks at Mission Hospital were my orientation. It was overwhelming, but I plugged away at it. During this time there were many small details to learn. Here in no particular order are the differences between the ways that a nurse works in a Mission Hospital in Nepal compared to a hospital in the US.

Gloves are recycled until they break. The gloves are latex. When they are soiled, the gloves are placed in a special bucket to be cleaned, re-powdered and recirculated. An employee of the supply department makes the rounds to collect the soiled gloves each day and bring a new supply.

The patient rooms do not have a sink. When the doctors make rounds, there is a special rolling hand washing station on a wheeled tripod that accompanies them so they can wash their hands between patients. The charge nurse reminds the doctors as if she is a mother nagging the kids. Near the nurse's station is a sink with a bar of soap and a fresh towel replenished each shift. All the nurses use the exact same pattern of systematic hand washing when they stand there, which ends by cupping water in the hands to splash over the faucet, almost as if for good luck.

At night, a family member brings in a bed roll and sleeps under the bed, awakening at two in the morning to measure and record their relatives' intake and output. If a patient is incontinent, the linen is changed by the family. At seven in the morning, the *Chowkidars* come and sweep through the wards, telling the relatives that they must leave for the two-hour period of doctors' and nurses' rounds. So as the employees arrive through the front gate, they are met by a stream of tired people carrying bedrolls.

Each unit has a Eurogard water purifier mounted on the wall, which plays a twinkly tune when water is flowing through it. There is only one water pitcher which is shared by all the staff, refilled from the Eurogard. There are no paper cups. All the Nepalis are experts at drinking straight from the pitcher without actually touching their lips to it. If a person's lips touch the pitcher, that breaks the rules of caste. The first ten times I tried this I spilled water over my scrub shirt.

Brahmins will only eat food prepared by other *Brahmins*. In the hospital neighborhood, there are more than dozen small hotels and each has a kitchen. These hotels cater to the families of patients, since many come great distances to get to Mission Hospital. The family will stay in a nearby hotel appropriate to their caste, and rely on the hotel staff to make *dal-bhaat*. At ten o'clock in the morning and again at six pm, there is a parade of families bringing *dal-bhaat* on covered stainless steel plates. The hospital does not provide food for the adult patients, unless they need a supplement, in which case they get *Sarbotham Pitto*. This is mainly grains with some vitamins added, and the staff would cook some over an open gas flame every morning. The smell of porridge now makes me think of mornings at the hospital, a sort of olfactory hallucination.

There is a *Hotel-Wallah* at each hotel. These men accompany the family members to the hospital and sometimes help the chaplains or the doctors with various tasks. The hotel neighborhood was given the name Shantytown many years ago, but then the Nepalis adapted the same name, because *Shanti* means peace in Nepali.

The usual time to give daily medications is one PM. The doctors write the name of the medication directly on the medication administration record and the nurses do not recopy the medication list. This is considerably simpler than the system most American hospitals use. Mission Hospital does not have a pharmacist in the Pharmacy department.

The medical staff only uses five antibiotics most of the time – gentamycin, ampicillin, penicillin, chloroamphenicol, and cefazolin. For adults, there is a standard dose for each one except the gentamycin. The nurse counts up the number of doses of ampicillin and reconstitutes them all at once, then does the same for the next antibiotic. The doses are piled on a single tray with one divider for each medication, not divided according to patient or room number. There are no trips back and forth to the medication preparation area once the nurse starts medication administration rounds. A checklist is used to indicate who gets what, but the individual syringes are not labeled with the drug name or individual names of patients. Most medications are given IV push. In the US, many antibiotics are given using a "piggyback" bag, but this system is less often used at Mission Hospital.

There are no IV pumps; everything is dripped and the drop rate is controlled by a hand roller on the IV line, the old fashioned way. Even dopamine, which is a powerful adrenergic drug, is given this way, with the added precaution of a "burette." As a rule, the patients have excellent veins – few people are obese. Many are manual laborers. It is easy to start an IV on a Nepali. No central lines and no PICC lines. The hospital does not yet have a needleless system. The nurses do not routinely wear gloves when handling IVs.

I rarely saw three-bottle chest drainage while I was there, and when it was needed they literally used three bottles on a little wheeled stand – no pleurevacs. Mostly they stuck to one drainage bag – strictly speaking, the "second bottle" of the three-bottle system. The first time I saw this I was skeptical. Surprisingly this system seems to meet most of the need for chest drainage.

The wooden beds are not adjustable. The beds are too close together to permit a stretcher in between, so when a patient needs to move from bed to stretcher the family does it or else we call the *peons* to come in a group of three and do a manual transfer. Sometimes relatives cry as they watch this. It was not until later that I learned the reason. When a person's body is cremated, three male relatives will lift it onto the pyre the exact same way. It triggers a memory. Women never attend a cremation in Tansen, by the way. Only men. By the same token, men never attend childbirth, not even if they are the father of the baby being born.

Nobody will get into bed between two white sheets, not for a million rupees. The sheets are blue or pink. White is the color of a shroud. There is space on the roof for clotheslines, and on sunny days baskets of wet sheets are carried up three flights of stairs and set out with clothespins. The hospital owns an industrial clothes dryer but only uses it during monsoon, to save electricity. The mattresses are about two inches thick, just like the ones at a typical Nepali home. Many people do not sleep on a mattress at home, just a woven mat.

The vast majority of newborn deliveries in our district take place at home. If the mother develops postpartum complications she is admitted to the Gynae Ward, not to the Maternity Ward. The Gynae Ward is an eleven-bed all-female "Nightingale style" open ward with drapes between. Babies are not given a name until eleven days of age. So the census lists them as "b/o Sanjita" or some such. b/o is short for "baby of..."

It is hard to find a piece of scrap paper. The charts include just the most important information. The hospital keeps the standard forms to a minimum, printed on cheap paper. If the patient is illiterate and needs to witness consent for an operation, there is an ink pad available so that a fingerprint can be used instead of a signature. When a patient is discharged, they are given their chart.

To get seen by a doctor in the ER or Outpatient Clinic, somebody has to go to the ticket window and buy a ticket. It must be paid for in cash before the doctor visit. There is a huge outpatient waiting room with long wooden benches. Downstairs from the main floor are separate clinics for leprosy, TB, and HIV disease, but there are many undiagnosed TB cases among the people sitting in the waiting area.

The Nursing Department of the Hospital is organized using a "functional nursing" model. Each employee starts the day with an assigned list of repetitive tasks. In other words, there is one nurse who gives all the medications, one nurse who takes all the blood pressures, one nurse who changes all the dressings. The only nurse who really has the Big Picture is the Charge Nurse or, *didi*. If you asked a staff nurse how they know when they are doing a better job, they would probably reply, "Because I can get the medications delivered more efficiently." This is in contrast to other models of care delivery that might be more conducive to an outcomes-oriented approach, where the nurse might reply, "Because my patients are improving faster with fewer complications."

The Nursing School is located just downhill from the Hospital, connected by a long straight stone staircase. The school is brick, constructed like a military fort with classrooms, offices and dorm space around a central plaza, guarded by its own *Chowkidars*. The students stay five-to-a-room, and the dorm rooms are smaller than my faculty office at UH. A student once told me that most of her classmates kept the same roommates for the entire three years of school. Restrooms and showers are at the end of the hall. The School has its own canteen, and if a student was on night duty she is allowed to appear in a track suit or something casual. When I ate at the canteen I enjoyed looking through the window to see the dozen or so goats owned by the School. The kitchen staff each take a turn at watching the goats, and every now and again a goat ends up in the mutton curry. As the main ingredient.

Students wear a uniform and old-fashioned nursing cap when at Clinical; on class days a bright purple *sari* with a white top, hair pulled back and no skin showing at the midriff. When the students cross the courtyard in their *saris*, it is like a flock of blue-and-white penguins going by. There are no male students. On Saturdays students are allowed to go the *Bajar* in western-style clothes. They are not allowed to have cell phones, a great hardship for teenage girls nowadays.

In the census book on the patient care floors, a column lists the caste of each person admitted. Nurses are very good at guessing caste without asking. At first I wondered why there were so many people with the last name " Bdr." Bdr is short for *Bahadur*, meaning that the patient is a Chhetri. Chhetris are the warrior caste, and *Bahadur* means "brave."

Appendix 5

Nepal Travel Warning

May 07, 2007

This Travel Warning provides updated information on the security situation in Nepal and notes the U.S. designation of the Communist Party of Nepal (Maoist) as a terrorist organization. The Department of State remains concerned about the security situation in Nepal and continues to urge American citizens contemplating a visit to Nepal to obtain updated security information before they travel and to be prepared to change their plans at short notice. This supersedes the Travel Warning issued on December 8, 2006.

Despite the signing of a comprehensive peace agreement by the Government and Maoist insurgents and their entry into an interim government, Maoists continue to engage in violence, extortion, and abductions. Maoists freely roam the countryside and cities, sometimes openly bearing their weapons. The Young Communist League, a subgroup of the Maoists, continues to extort and abuse people, including threatening Kathmandu-based personnel of a U.S. Non Governmental Organization. Maoist leader Puspa Dahal (aka "Prachanda") publicly alleged in March 2007 that royalists were planning to assassinate U.S. government personnel, but Dahal never offered any evidence for his claim. Furthermore, in a May 1, 2007 speech, Dahal threatened to launch a new campaign of demonstrations and disruptions.

Violent clashes between Maoists and indigenous groups have taken place in recent months in the *Terai* region, along the southern border with India, in one case resulting in 27 deaths. Ethnic tensions in the Terai region have spawned violent clashes with police, strikes, demonstrations and closures of the border with India. The U.S. Embassy strongly recommends against non-essential travel to this region. Clashes between Maoists and groups who oppose them also recently have extended into Kathmandu.

In November 2006 numerous resident American citizens reported to the U.S. Embassy first-hand accounts of Maoist cadres demanding food and lodging, often accompanied by threats of physical violence. In some instances, Nepalese staff of Americans who resisted such demands were beaten. Since the cease-fire in May 2006, hotels and businesses frequented by American citizens have been targets of extortion demands, forced closures, and have become the focus of demonstrations. While widespread protests have abated, the potential for demonstrations and disruptions remains high. During demonstrations, protestors have used violence, including burning vehicles, throwing rocks and burning tires to block traffic. Given the nature, intensity and unpredictability of disturbances, American citizens are urged to exercise special caution during times when demonstrations are announced, avoid areas where demonstrations are occurring or crowds are forming, avoid road travel, and maintain a low profile. Curfews can be announced with little or no advance notice, and American citizens are urged to consult media sources and the Embassy's website (nepal.usembassy.gov) for current security information.

Crime in the Kathmandu Valley, including violent crime and harassment of women, has increased since April 2006. Travel via road in areas outside of the Kathmandu valley is still dangerous and should be avoided. Police have reported a number of robberies by armed gangs; in some cases victims were attacked and injured. The U.S. Embassy reports an increase in crime in some popular tourist areas. Visitors to Nepal should practice good personal security when moving about, especially at night, and avoid walking alone after dark and carrying large sums of cash or wearing expensive jewelry. In several reported incidents tourists have had their belongings stolen from their rooms while they were asleep. In late 2005, two European women were murdered in Nargarjun Forest, a popular tourist destination in the Kathmandu Valley. The murders occurred within weeks of each other and both involved women hiking alone. In March 2006, Maoists detained several Polish trekkers after the trekkers refused to pay extortion. Solo trekkers have been robbed by small groups of young men, even on some popular trails. Crime, including violent crime, has further increased in 2007, and police are unwilling or unable to arrest criminals who claim Maoist affiliation.

U.S. official personnel generally do not travel by road outside the Kathmandu Valley. All official travel outside the Kathmandu valley, including by air, requires specific clearance by the U.S. Embassy's Regional Security Officer. As a result, emergency assistance to U.S. citizens may be limited. Active duty U.S. military and Department of Defense contractors must obtain a country clearance for official and unofficial travel to Nepal.

Although the Government of Nepal no longer considers the Maoists to be terrorists, the U.S. government's designation of the Communist Party of Nepal (Maoist) as a "Specially Designated Global Terrorist" organization under Executive Order 13224 and its inclusion on the "Terrorist Exclusion List" pursuant to the Immigration and Nationality Act remain in effect. These two designations make Maoists excludable from entry into the United States and bar U.S. citizens from transactions such as contribution of funds, goods, or services to, or for the benefit of, the Maoists.

U.S. citizens who travel to or reside in Nepal are urged to register with the Consular Section of the Embassy by accessing the Department of State's travel registration site at travelregistration.state.gov or by personal appearance at the Consular Section, located at the Yak and Yeti Hotel complex just east of Durbarmarg Street. The Consular Section can provide updated information on travel and security, and can be phoned directly at (977) (1) 444-5577 or through the Embassy switchboard. The U.S. Embassy is located at Pani Pokhari in Kathmandu, telephone (977) (1) 441-1179; fax (977) (1) 444-4981, website: nepal.usembassy.gov.

U.S. citizens also should consult the Department of State's Consular Information Sheet for Nepal and Worldwide Caution Public Announcement via the Internet on the Department of State's home page at travel.state.gov or by calling 1-888-407-4747 toll free in the United States and Canada, or, for callers outside the United States and Canada, a regular toll line at 1-202-501-4444. These numbers are available from 8:00 a.m. to 8:00 p.m. Eastern Time, Monday through Friday (except U.S. federal holidays).

Appendix 6

Jesus Prays on the Mount of Olives

Luke 22

39 Jesus went out as usual to the Mount of Olives, and his disciples followed him. 40 On reaching the place, he said to them, "Pray that you will not fall into temptation." 41 He withdrew about a stone's throw beyond them, knelt down and prayed, 42 "Father, if you are willing, take this cup from me; yet not my will, but yours be done." 43 An angel from heaven appeared to him and strengthened him. 44 And being in anguish, he prayed more earnestly, and his sweat was like drops of blood falling to the ground.

45 When he rose from prayer and went back to the disciples, he found them asleep, exhausted from sorrow. 46 "Why are you sleeping?" he asked them. "Get up and pray so that you will not fall into temptation."

Mark 14

32 And they came to a place which was named Gethsemane: and he saith to his disciples, Sit ye here, while I shall pray. 33 And he taketh with him Peter and James and John, and began to be sore amazed, and to be very heavy; 34 And saith unto them, My soul is exceeding sorrowful unto death: tarry ye here, and watch. 35 And he went forward a little, and fell on the ground, and prayed that, if it were possible, the hour might pass from him. 36 And he said, Abba, Father, all things are possible unto thee; take away this cup from me: nevertheless not what I will, but what thou wilt. 37 And he cometh, and findeth them sleeping, and saith unto Peter, Simon, sleepest thou? couldest not thou watch one hour? 38 Watch ye and pray, lest ye enter into temptation. The spirit truly is ready, but the flesh is weak. 39 And again he went away, and prayed, and spake the same words. 40 And when he returned, he found them asleep again, (for their eyes were heavy,) neither wist they what to answer him. 41 And he cometh the third time, and saith unto them, Sleep on now, and take your rest: it is enough, the hour is come; behold, the Son of man is betrayed into the hands of sinners.

Confirmed Birds

Pied Cukoo (clamator Jacobinus)
Black Kite (milvus migrans)
Oriental honey buzzard (pernis ptilorhynus)
House Crow (corvus splendus)
Whiterumped Shama(copsychus malabricus)
Wiretailed Swallow (hirundo smithii)
Red-vented Bulbul (alophoixus flaveolus)
Common Mynah (acridotherus tristis)

Bibliography

Cocker, Dorothy. *Aids to Tropical Nursing.* Bailliere, Tindall and Cox, London, 1959.

Cook, J., Sankaran, B., Wasunna, E.A.O. *Surgery at the District Hospital.* World Health Organization, 1988.

Hull, Eleanor; *Be Thou My Vision.* Song, traditional. Original lyrics by Forgaill, Dallan, 8th century. current verse 1912.

Grimmett, Richard; Inskipp, Carol; and Inskipp, Tim. *Princeton Field Guides: Birds of Nepal.* Princeton University Press, 2000.

Hale,Thomas. *On Being a Missionary.* William Carey Library, Pasadena California, 1995.

Hockenberry, Marilyn; Wilson, David. *Wong's Nursing Care of Infants and Children.* 6th edition, Mosby, St Louis 2006.

Khadka, Rajendra (editor). *Traveler's Tales NEPAL True Stories of Life on the Road.* Traveler's Tales, San Francisco, 1997.

McHugh, Ernestine. *Love and Honor in the Himalayas.* (Contemporary Ethnography Series), Cornell University Press, April 2001.

Mindrolling Jetsun Khandro. *37 Practices of a Boddhisattva.* Public Lectures at Kagyu Thegchen Ling, Honolulu Tibetan Monastery, October 2006, www.vkr.org. www.vkr.org.

Moran, Kerry. *NEPAL.* 4th edition, Moon Handbooks, Avalon Travel, 2004, moon.com.

Rinchen, Geshe Sonam. *Thirty Seven Practices of a Boddhisattva.* Snow Lion Publications, Ithaca, New York, 1997

Schull, Christopher R. *Common Medical Problems in the Tropics.* 2nd edition, MacMillan Publishers, London and Oxford, 1999,talcuk. com.

Sehlinger, Bob. *Unofficial Guide to Disney World.* MacMillan, (annually updated), 1999

Martin, Max; Carlssen, Andreas. *Tell Me Why.* Backstreet Boys, Millenium, 1999.

Thompson, Hunter S. Fear and Loathing in Las Vegas, 2nd edition, Vintage, 1998 originally published in Rolling Stone, 1971

US State Department Travel advisory travel.state.gov/travel/cis_pa_tw/ cis/cis_980.hthm

Glossary of Nepali Terms

These are included for the reader's convenience. This is not an all-inclusive lexicon, but does show Nepali words in common use among English-speaking foreigners in Tansen.

Achaar – the Nepali equivalent of Ketchup. A condiment served as a side dish to rice and lentil soup. There are many subtle variations of spice which make it the bright point of dhal-bhaat.

Auz, Aussie – from Australia.

Bajar – "Bazaar". The marketplace of a town, with open-fronted specialty shops.

Batch – group or cohort. This is the term for a graduating class, used throughout Nepal.

Bhandh – literally "closed." The term used for any work stoppage, esp. if politically inspired. A frequent occurrence.

Bhangra – a form of pop music with videos, made in Bombay, similar to MTV in the USA.

Brahmin – an upper-caste Nepali.

Buff – short for Buffalo. A type of meat served in lieu of beef.

Carom – a board game that uses disks shaped like checkers and is played like billiards.

Chapattis – flat bread, usually cooked in a clay oven. Also called "roti".

Cheroot – a tobacco cigarette.

Chhetri – the warrior caste, similar to Brahmins, of Aryan origin, light-skinned.

Chiya – Nepali tea made by boiling the leaves and milk with the water then strained. Strong.

Cholo – double-breasted blouse worn by Magar women. Similar to a Tibetan design but heavier cloth is used.

Chowkidar – security guard. At Mission Hospital most of these were Muslims.

Dankini – a supernatural creature, feminine in nature, which can invade your body. Periodically, the gods will come down and fight against hordes of malevolent dankinis.

Dhaka – hand-woven cloth with colorful designs made in Tansen and vicinity.

Devanagari – the script used in written Nepali, similar to Sanskrit. A "syllabary" as opposed to an "alphabet".

Dhara – water source. Sometimes a stream, sometimes a tap, sometimes a faucet mounted in a wall, sometimes a tank.

Dal-bhaat – the daily meal of the average Nepali. Cooked rice served with a small dish of lentil soup which is poured over the rice and eaten with the fingers of the right hand.

Didi – "older sister" or a female servant. Used literally to address any woman older than you.

Dokaa – a bamboo pack basket used by Magars which also uses a tumpline.

Durbar – a palace or grand building.

Ganesh – The Hindu god, son of Shiva, with the elephant's head. Known as "the remover of obstacles." Before you pray to any other God, you ask Ganesh to help make your prayers effective.

Ghat – a stone platform from which cremations are carried out. When the fire is done the ashes are shoveled into a nearby river.

Gurhka – member of one of the Nepal mercenary regiments that served with the UK military. Fierce fighters.

Gurung – an ethnic group related to the Magars. More prominent in the Annapurna region. Home of the Gurkhas.

Hajur – the honorific term for a person of higher social standing than you, translated as "sir".

Honorific – technical linguistic term used in language instruction, for a verb tense which implies awareness of relative social status when addressing a person of superior rank or caste.

Janai – a cord worn around the waist or shoulder of a devout Brahmin.

Jeevan Jal – the trade name for the commonly used solution in oral rehydration therapy. It comes in powdered form and is added to filtered water. Given to patients with diarrhea.

Kala-Azar – Nepali name for Visceral Leishmaniasis, an illness spread using dogs and sandworms as intermediary vectors.

Kama Sutra – a book of eroticism from Medieval India. Imaginative use of positions. Be sure to check out page 42!

Kata – a white scarf used as a blessing.

Ke garne? – An expression of fatalism "what is there that can be done?"

Khukri – a large knife used in Nepal, with a distinctive shape, carried by the Gurkhas as a weapon for hand-to-hand fighting.

Krait – *Bungarus Fasciatus*, a poisonous snake. Venom is up to sixteen times more lethal than that of the cobra. Can grow up to four feet long, the diameter of a broomstick. Nocturnal.

Kurtha Surwal – clothing item of many Nepali women.

Lathi – a four foot long bamboo stick used as a weapon.

Lungi – a wraparound gown, loose fitting and ankle length. In the case of men from the Terai, characteristically blue plaid.

Magar – name of a large ethnic group. Reputation for honesty and work ethic.

Missionary Position – woman on back, man on top, both horizontal.

Maoists – not related to the Chinese. Political party which spearheaded the Nepal civil war (1992-2004).

Mehandi lagaunu – to put henna on your hands, during summer.

Mojo – (not a Nepali word.) libido, the momentum of manliness. Slang of African-American origin. Originally, a magic charm consisting of a red flannel bag with botanical substances in it, worn under the clothes, conveys special powers to the wearer.

Momo – Tibetan food dish, small bits of meat wrapped in pastry and steamed or fried.

Monkey – monkeys described in this book are the "Rhesus Macaque," *Macaca mulatta*, found throughout South Asia.

Mutton – the euphemism for goat meat. Be sure to pronounce *both* "Ts"

"Namaste" – a greeting and a farewell both. Accompanied by a specific gesture. Sometimes shortened in to a low "tayyyyyy".

Newari – tribe of Nepalis mostly found in Kathmandu. Merchants and traders.

NGO – Non-Governmental Organization, usually an international charity of some kind.

Oz – Australia (slang).

Pashmina – belly wool of a Nepali goat. Highly prized fiber for shawls.

Patuka – wraparound belt of a Magar woman. Five meters long.

Phewa Tal – lake in Pokhara, sometimes transliterated "Taal"

Potey – green beaded necklace the color of new rice shoots.

Proms – in London England, a series of summer concerts in the outdoors, short for "Promenades," the last night of which is given over to nostalgia and patriotic tunes.

Puja – Hindu or Buddhist prayer ceremony, usually accompanied by an offering.

Pugio – literally "reached." the term used to indicate that you no longer want a refill of dal-bhaat. Or that you are finished with something.

Pulchowk – a neighborhood of Patan.

Raksi – homemade alcohol. Distilling equipment for this purpose was sold in every hardware store.

Rinpoche – In Tibetan Buddhism, a person with a documented history of reincarnation.

Sadhu – a Hindu holy man who has renounced material possessions.

Samosa – a food item made of vegetables wrapped in flaky dough and deep-fried.

Sangha – (one of the three pillars of Buddhism, along with Buddha and Dharma.) Refers to the cohort of people with whom you go through any given cycle of your existence. Used to colloquially to mean "friend".

Sar – the Nepali pronunciation of "Sir".

Sarbotham Pitto – a nutritional supplement composed of high-protein grains and vitamins, smells like porridge, widely used in lesser developed countries.

Sari – clothing item, consisting of six meters of cloth.

Shiva – "the destroyer," a major Hindu deity, patron of Pashupattinath.

Stupa – a ceremonial mound which is a place of Buddhist worship.

Tantric path – A form of mystical Buddhist practice which does not rely on logic, but is experiential in nature. Often associated with sexual practices but the term applies to many situations.

Terai – the low lying valley on the border with India, hot and humid, rice-growing region, former jungle with endemic malaria.

Teva ® – brand name of a type of sandal used by outdoors persons, (not a Nepali word).

Thapa – the name given by Brahmins and Chhetris to the persons of Asian descent such as the Magars.

Theater – British term for the Operating Room.

Thik cha – Nepali phrase meaning "okay".

Thrash, thrashing – specifically, frontier justice administered by a committee or posse of citizens with bamboo lathis, as opposed to a mere beating. Simplifies the need for court proceedings.

Tika – the little mark which covers the "third eye" or sixth chakra. Indicates Hinduism.

Toot – short for "tutorial."

Topi – a) the cap worn by men b) the knot of hair left after a ritual haircut at a funeral.

Torch – flashlight.

Tigers and Goats (bagh-chal) a popular board game in Nepal.

Trek – a guided hike in the mountains, usually accompanied by porters who carry everything for you. The main tourist industry of Nepal.

Tuk-Tuk – a small three-wheeled motorized vehicle used for cheap transportation in Kathmandu and other large Asian cities. The ones in Nepal are larger than the ones in Thailand or Vietnam.

Tundikhel – large flat field used as a parade ground.

UMN – United Missions to Nepal – an international Christian NGO of world churches active in Nepal since 1952.

Videshi – foreigner.

Wallah – (always a suffix, never a standalone word) the owner of some entrepreneurial enterprise, such as a hotel. A big fish in some small pond.

Westerner – non-Nepali; anybody from a "G-8 country," dressed like an obvious tourist.

Translations of Book Jacket Comments

As an experienced nurse (previously in Nepal and currently in USA), I can attest that this book is a realistic portrayal of hospital care in Nepal. I worked in many hospitals in Nepal but the challenges were similar and the author vividly shows a typical day in any hospital in Nepal.

Mandira Aryal Neupane, RN (California and Hawaii)
(Ms Neupane is currently working at Straub Clinic and Hospital, Honolulu, HI)

एउटा अनुभबी नर्स (पहीले नेपालमा र हाल अमेरीकामा कार्यरत) को आधारमा म नौर्धक्क संग के भन्न सक्दछु भने यस पुस्तकले नेपालको अस्पताल सेवा लाई स्पष्ट चीत्रण गर्दछ | मेरो अनुभबमा नेपालका धेरै अस्पतालहरुमा एकै कीसीमका समस्याहरु छन् र लेखक ले नेपालको कुनै पनी अस्पतालमा दैनीक रुपमा हुनसक्ने परीस्थीती लाई राम्रोसंग प्रस्तुत गरेका छन |

मन्दीरा अर्याल न्यौपाने, आर एन (क्यालीफोर्नीया र हवाई)
(श्रीमती न्यौपाने हाल स्टरब क्लीनीक एण्ड हस्पटिल होनोलुलु हवाईमा कार्यरत हुनुहुन्छ।)

In this book author Joe Niemczura presents the experiences he gained when he worked in Tansen Mission Hospital as a volunteer health worker. Niemczura has given a good introduction on how sincerely Nepalese and foreign health workers meet daily challenges to address numerous and difficult cases with limited and often antiquated resources. Much more than a dry account of problems of health services in rural Nepal, this book embodies true and fascinating narrative that keeps the reader entertained.

Dr. Alok Rajouria

यस पुस्तकमा लेखक जो नीम्ज्राले तानसेन मीसन हस्पीटलमा स्वयं सेवक सुवास्थकर्मीका रुपमा संगालेका अनुभवहरु प्रस्तुत गरेका छन् । नीम्ज्राले वीवीध तथा जटील समस्याहरु लीएर आउने बीरामीहरुको सेवामा समर्पीत नेपाली तथा बीदेशी स्वास्थकर्मीहरुले दैनीक सामना गर्नुपर्ने चुनौतीहरुको राम्रो परीचय दीएकाछन । नेपालको दुर्गम ग्रामीण जीबनमा आईपर्ने सुवास्थ सेवाका समस्याहरुको रुखो बर्णन नभई यो एक यथार्थपूर्ण र रोचक बृतान्त हो जसले पाठकलाई रोमान्चीत तुल्याउछ |
डा. आलोक रजौरीया डा. रजौरीया, एक अर्थ तथा समाज शास्तुरी, हाल युनीभर्सीटी अफ हवाई मा कार्यरत छन् ।

258

About the Author

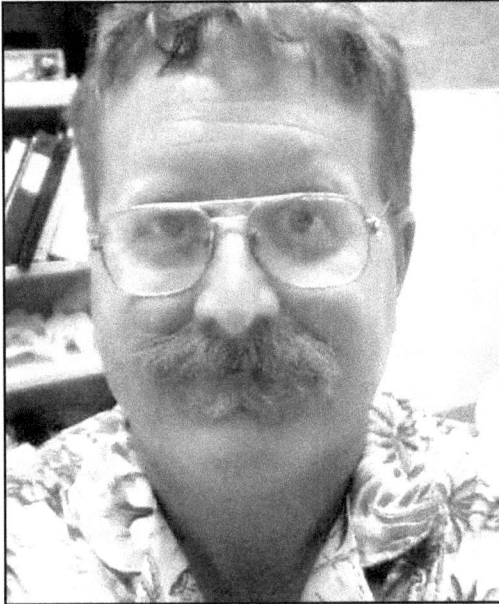

Joe Niemczura now teaches nursing at the University of Hawaii at Manoa. He holds nursing degrees from the University of Massachusetts at Amherst (BS, 1977) and the University of California at San Francisco (MS, 1981). He has been active with the American Nurses Association, and is a past President of ANA-Maine, where he lived for nearly thirty years. He has never regretted his choice of career. His younger daughter is a teacher, gardener, and poet; the older daughter is a linguist, and traveler. He enjoys living in Honolulu where there are no snakes and it is warm enough to wear slippers year-round.

Contact the author at joeniemczura@gmail.com. Also find *The Hospital At the End of the World* on Facebook to see more photos, videos and other background information.

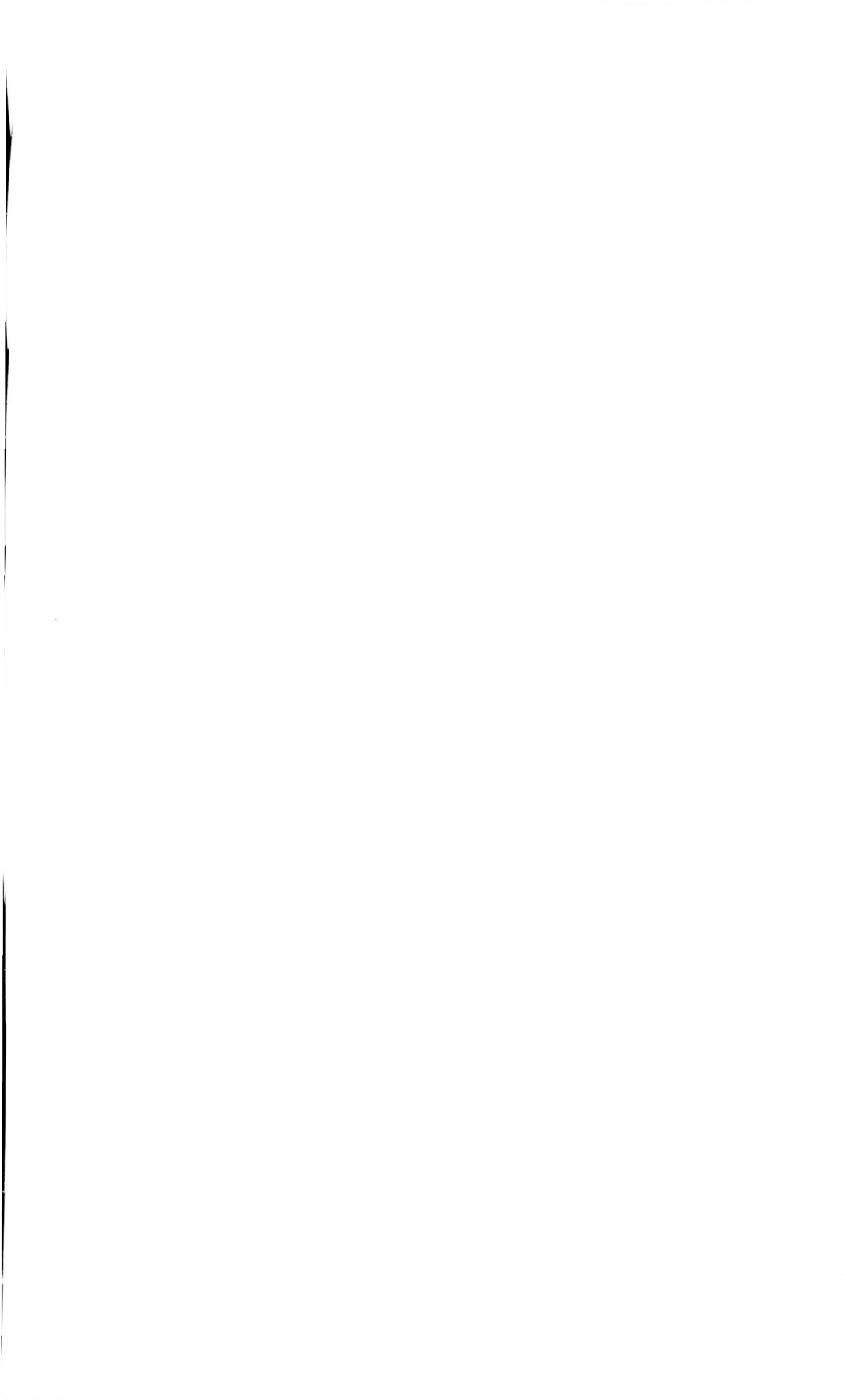